"**GREAT SHAPE** contains all the magic, encouragement, and self-love possible in 272 pages. . . . They write with a sparkle that energized me, a consciousness that awed me, and a compassion that touched me."

Nancy Barron, Ph.D.
Director, Ample Opportunity

"**This book** could be called 'The Joy of Moving!' Packed with saavy for women of all sizes and ages."

Sadja Greenwood, M.D.
Co-author, *The Medical Self-Care Book of Women's Health*

"**A superb book** that jogs professional minds to a liberating new paradigm where health, not weight loss, is the goal."

Laura Keranen, M.P.H.
Director, Health Education
Kaiser Permanente, Northern California

"**As a Registered Dietitian** specializing in the area of obesity, I found this book an invaluable tool for helping larger women become more active. I especially appreciated the photos of large women enjoying themselves hiking, swimming, playing tennis, doing karate, weight lifting and aerobic dancing. These are women my clientele can identify with and model themselves after! The book proves that being large does not have to result in a sedentary lifestyle."

Joanne Ikeda, M.A., R.D.
Extension Nutrition Education Specialist
University of California
Author of *Winning Weight Loss For Teens*

"**It's GREAT!!!** I'm really impressed with the information and the way it's presented. I especially like the combination of presenting factual information and personal experience."

Jane M. Moore, Ph.D., R.D.
Nutrition Consultant
Oregon State Health Division

"**GREAT SHAPE** is for everyone, no matter what size of large. The clothing resources in the appendix are worth the price of the book."

Frances White
Board of Directors
National Association to Advance Fat
Acceptance

"**Building on the too-true premise** that the overweight are discouraged from exercise and sports participation, the authors (large and lovely themselves) simultaneously encourage and instruct. . . . Finally, there is a voice in the fitness wilderness saying what we all need to hear: 'You're okay.'"
Booklist

"**Espousing the philosophy** that 'fat and fit are not mutually exclusive,' the authors offer welcome encouragement to their fellow large women. . . . Some advice has wider application and will appeal to anyone battling the 'couch-potato' and 'no time, no money' syndromes, fear of failure or injury, or the still-extant problems of competing in games traditionally considered 'male only.'"
Publishers Weekly

"**Their descriptions** of various sports and forms of exercise—softball, skiing, walking, bicycling, etc.—are often lyrical, and should entice even sedentary women to get moving. A real boost: many of the aerobic dance steps and calisthenic routines have been modified so that heavier women can perform them without risk of injury to bone or muscle."
Kirkus Reviews

"**GREAT SHAPE** is motivating and packed with sound information about every facet of exercise, from safety to finding large size exercise clothing."
Medical SelfCare Magazine

". . . **a great book** about movement and health for large women. Solidly feminist in approach, content and philosophy . . ."
The Feminist Bookstore News

". . . **their book help[s]** the larger-sized participant. . . . to overcome feelings of embarrassment and anxiety when facing exercise, and explain[s] how to get and stay involved in physical activities."
IDEA Today

". . . **the best book** of its kind that I have ever read."
Pacific Sun (Mill Valley, CA)

"**For women** who are naturally large, GREAT SHAPE will be a welcome change from the normal exercise book aimed at making you slim and trim regardless of your natural physique and the personal physical cost in trying to trim it down."
Abilene Reporter-News (Abilene, Texas)

GREAT SHAPE

GREAT SHAPE

THE FIRST
FITNESS GUIDE
FOR LARGE WOMEN

PAT LYONS AND DEBBY BURGARD

AN AUTHORS GUILD BACKINPRINT.COM EDITION

Great Shape:
The First Fitness Guide For Large Women
All Rights Reserved © 1988, 2000 by Patricia A. Lyons and Debora L. Burgard

AN AUTHORS GUILD BACKINPRINT.COM EDITION

Published by iUniverse.com, Inc.

For information address:
iUniverse.com, Inc.
620 North 48th Street, Suite 201
Lincoln, NE 68504-3467
www.iuniverse.com

Originally published by Morrow

ISBN: 0-595-08883-X

Printed in the United States of America

———————————————————————— ▰▰ ————————————————————————

"Loves music. Loves dance. Loves the moon. Loves the Spirit. Loves love and food and roundness. Loves struggle. Loves the Folk. Loves herself. Regardless."

Alice Walker defining a "womanist," from
In Search of Our Mothers' Gardens

Table of Contents

Acknowledgements xi
Preface xv
Introduction xvii

Chapter 1   **Fat and Fit   1**
An Idea Whose Time Has Come

Chapter 2   **Getting Started   25**
A Different Approach

Chapter 3   **Exercise and Weight   36**
Separating Fact from Propaganda

Chapter 4   **Warm-ups, Cool-downs, and Stretches   58**

Chapter 5   ***We Dance* Exercises and Dance Steps   75**

Chapter 6   **I'd Walk a Mile for a Swim   101**
Walking and Swimming for No Pain, All Gain

Chapter 7   **Sports for Any Body (Yes, This Means You)   126**

Chapter 8   **Learning Body Awareness   145**
Tips from Sport Psychology

Chapter 9   **Pitfalls, Detours, Comebacks   168**
How to Keep Yourself Motivated

Appendix I   **Annotated Bibliography   189**

Books
Magazines/Newsletters
Additional Relevant Research

Appendix II   **Exercise Resources   199**

Classes
Organizations
Exercise Videos/Review of the Exercise Videos

Appendix III   **Clothing   217**

Clothing Resources
Review of the Dancewear
Sewing Resources

Appendix IV   **Becoming an Instructor   227**

Appendix V   **For Instructors: Starting a Class for Large
Women   231**

Index 237

Acknowledgments

This book was simply meant to be. The basic premise—that fat and fit are not mutually exclusive terms—was the heart of my master's thesis. Debby and I had been acting on this premise in our different professional arenas for some time before we met, and through a series of serendipitous events we discovered each other and started working together to bring this unconventional idea to you.

When my thesis was finished I began wondering how I might translate its ideas into a popular book. I came across an article in *Ms.* magazine by Carol Sternhell entitled "We May Always Be Fat, but Fat Can Be Fit." Uh-oh. It was a great article, but a wave of anxiety came over me: If I didn't write my book immediately, someone else would! So I stared at my telephone. I could call *Ms.*, find out Carol's address, write to her and ask if she was writing *my* book, and if so, I could stop dreaming about myself as an author and get on with other things.

I dialed, despite the butterflies in my stomach. No, they couldn't give me her address, but the woman who answered suggested I call her at New York University where she teaches journalism. Well, what the hell. I got the number, dialed, and when she came on the line I sort of stammered and told her how much I liked her article. She was appreciative but slightly suspicious: "Surely you didn't call me just to tell me you love my writing."

"Well, in fact, I've been thinking about writing a book on 'fat and fit' and I was just wondering if you were intending to do so too," I said and held my breath. "No," she said. "Exercise is not really my thing, but a literary agent called me earlier today with just that question. I can give you her number."

After thanking her and hanging up I sat there sort of stunned. Go ahead, call the agent, said a bold and fearless voice in my head. This being my day for leaps of faith, I called. And to make a long story short, here we are!

Our thanks to the woman from *Ms.* who referred me to Carol, to Carol for her inspiring article and the referral to agent Eileen Fallon, to Eileen for her belief in this work and selling the proposal to Arbor House, and to editors Sarah Williamson, Beth Rashbaum, and Liza Dawson for being willing to take a chance on a book that didn't promise another "miracle weight loss plan."

This book could not have been conceived without the work of all the large people and their allies working for size acceptance who have come before us. We thank the Fat Underground, Fat Chance, the National Association to Advance Fat Acceptance (NAAFA), and Fat Lip Readers' Theater for defining and discussing the health and social issues of fat women long before the medical establishment would listen. It is these groups who have paved the road to self-acceptance for all large women through their art and consciousness-raising.

Alice Ansfield, publisher of *Radiance: The Magazine for Large Women,* deserves our special thanks for carrying the pioneering work of the above groups forward and publishing our ideas in *Radiance* so they could be shared with a national audience. Thanks to Eliza Mimsky, who taught the first "fat and fit" class in San Francisco, and to Rosezella Canty-Letsome, who encouraged us from the start.

Many women, some of whom are quoted or pictured in the book, believed in us, provided us with insights, and inspired us by being living proof that large women can be strong, courageous, healthy, witty—and fun to play with! Thanks to the We Dancers: Rosemary Senegal, Peggy Wilson, Robin Hopkins, Carol Squires, Frances White, Cheryl White, Ruth Lafler, Gloria Law, Darolyn Maker, Renee Brooks, Eleanor Walker, and all the other women who have danced their way through the class over the years. Thanks to all the women from the "Making Waves" Saturday swim, especially Miriam Cantor and Sandy Shepherd; and to the other sporting women: Danita Kulp, Linda Minor, Michelle Dethke, Taree Lyn Klausner, Terri Ramey, Rita Northrop Jones, Margaret Orlando, Cheron Dudley, Carol Thomas, and Bettye Travis.

Special thanks to Robin Hopkins and Frances White for researching the clothing resources, and to Lee Eastman for sharing her personal story. Thanks to Kerry Tegman of Flying Foxes for providing our models with beautiful leotards. Robin Dochterman of the Women's Sports Foundation provided us with statistics on the participation of women in sports, and the Foundation itself deserves ample recognition for leading the movement toward equality in sports for women and girls.

Our photographer Irene Young was a crucial partner in this venture, bringing forth our vision of the beauty and strength of large women having a great time. We also thank Mary Aldridge for sharing her expertise in exercise physiology.

Pat's personal thanks go to Harry Edwards, whose brilliance as a teacher and fierce courage to expose both racism and sexism in the world of sport inspired me to stay true to my principles despite their unpopularity; to American Indian women who showed me over and over that large women can be great athletes and who helped me realize that all oppression must be addressed before any of us can be free; to Maggie, Kathy, and Goldie for their constant support and friendship, and to Mom for knowing that my life would be richer if I was active in sports and for making that possible from the beginning.

Debby's personal thanks go to my teachers in African dance who inspired my awe and joyfully drew forth the dancer hiding in me; to the movement therapists at Feeding Ourselves and Tonda Thomas for planting the seed of We Dance in my head; and to my family, friends, co-workers, and Jeff for their unflagging love and support. I thank my We Dance and Dance Boogie students for the daily miracle of their blooming. Finally, I thank Pat for putting up with me even after she found out about my deep trouble with procrastination! It has been a heartfelt and rich collaboration.

Preface

Great Shape is the first fitness book written by and for large women. We are thrilled to have it back in print, and thank the Author's Guild for making this possible. We also want to thank the thousands of large women, supportive health professionals, and others who have joined us in the Health at Every Size revolution of the 90's. Fat prejudice is still alive and well. At the same time, Camryn Manheim won an Emmy for her role in "The Practice" and exuberantly dedicated it "to all the fat girls!" Large women are dancing, playing and enjoying life just as we are. No more waiting! So if you're still on the sidelines, we invite you to jump in.

It's Been the Best of Times…And the Worst of Times

Although we've each spent the past several years practicing in different healthcare settings, we still share a love of sport, dance and movement. We have not wavered in our belief that the purpose of movement is pleasure and enjoyment, not weight loss. We have seen over and over that health, self-esteem and body confidence can improve independently of changes in weight. We also share a professional commitment to improve the health and well-being of women of all sizes who are struggling in a culture that now worships even smaller 'heroin chic' waif models and media stars. Where a size 6 used to be considered thin enough, size 0 is now on clothing racks. While our focus in this book is on movement, not food and eating, we continue to encourage all women to stop dieting as a critical step in the process of improving health. Dieting, deprivation and self-hatred are problems, not solutions. There are many excellent books and counselors who can guide you in the process of ending the dieting cycle. Sound nutrition and healthy eating—which includes enjoying eating as one of life's pleasures—is for people of all sizes. And so is fitness.

We were the first to publish the idea that people could be both 'fat and fit' because it was true for us and for the other women you'll meet in these pages. In the Great Shape Program that Pat and Laura Keranen developed at Kaiser Permanente in Northern California from 1989-1997, large women instructors led more than 1500 women to better health. Women of all ages danced, stretched, laughed, and supported each other in trying this new approach. In program evaluation, women reported feeling better in many ways, including improvements in everyday strength and endurance, as well as in blood pressure or diabetes in those with such conditions. Women spoke of being less depressed, more optimistic and willing to try new things. For many, eating more fruits and vegetables replaced focusing on what not to eat. Discussions about how to cope with daily insults were interspersed with practice in "just saying no" to being weighed at every medical visit. Women who had refused to settle for negative experiences with medical care encouraged others to keep looking for a health care provider who would treat them with respect. While some women lost a few pounds, weight was not officially measured, and there were no dramatic "before" and "after" pictures. The focus was on living healthfully now. Many women found their doctors to be very supportive. One woman said: "My doctor told me, 'Whatever you're doing, keep it up'—so here I am!"

Several research studies published in the last few years have also demonstrated that 'fat and fit' is not fantasy. Studies conducted with thousands of people by Dr. Steven Blair and his colleagues at the Cooper Institute for Aerobic Research in Dallas have consistently demonstrated health benefits of being physically active that are independent of weight. One study found that "normal weight" men whose who were unfit had a death rate three times higher than fat men who were fit. As chief editor of the U.S. Surgeon General's report, *Physical Activity and Health,* Blair is a strong voice in the effort to make shame-free gyms, playgrounds, sports and fitness programs available to children and adults of all sizes. Research demonstrating that some activity is much better than none, and that you don't have to become a marathon runner to obtain health benefits, resulted in new activity recommendations from the federal Centers for Disease Control and Prevention. They now advise that 30 minutes of moderate activity on most days—anything from gardening, to taking the stairs instead of the elevator, to 10-minute walks around the block—

pays off in big health benefits. And they also recommend having fun because you're more likely to stick with it.

Well, it's just so tempting to say: We told you so. It's even tempting to think that we played a part in all of this. In 1988 when we first published many of these ideas, we were called radical, fresh, progressive, cutting edge. But of course, many people also called us crazy. Some people got really angry that we would even suggest such ideas! While we have experienced great readiness and enthusiasm for our ideas all along, here at the start of the new millennium we are still considered radical to some. Amazing that there is such resistance to an idea that just seems like common sense to us: *Fitness and health are for every body.*

We could add chapters covering new research studies in the fields of genetics, exercise science, nutrition, psychology, mind-body neuroscience, social support and public health that support our point of view even more strongly now. We are also very aware of newspaper headlines trumpeting a so-called "obesity epidemic." There is still plenty of disagreement about whether obesity is even a disease. Setting that debate aside, it is true that despite the billions that Americans have spent annually in weight loss efforts, more people are heavier than ever. But to this day, no weight loss treatment program has evidence that they beat the 5% long-term "success" rates reported at the 1992 National Institutes of Health meetings. Even though study after study has found that no matter what people try (particularly if they try to lose more than 10% of their body weight), the vast majority regain weight within 2-5 years. But these same treatments are still conducted at hospitals, clinics, and other locations all over the world.

We happen to be among those who believe that dieting and weight loss treatment—with its almost inevitable weight regain—has, in fact, been a significant factor in the increased numbers of people who are now heavier. And Debby consistently points out to her colleagues treating eating disorders that what is *diagnosed* as disordered eating in thin people is what is *prescribed* for fat people! Clients in standard weight management programs are told to put weight loss at the center of their life; to see fat as bad and getting thinner as good; to relentlessly monitor fat grams, calories and minutes of exercise; to avoid people and social gatherings that might make them 'go off their program'; and to use the scale as their main measurement of success.

Well, as the old adage goes: Follow the money. The diet industry continues to rake in billions in profits, while drug companies cash in on society's hunger for the next new miracle diet pill. The Redux

/Phen-Fen diet pill disaster and subsequent drug recall has not stopped the FDA from approving other drugs with significant risks and little benefit to show for such risks. (Where are those 'just say no to drugs' people when we really need them?) And perhaps you were among the 29 million Americans who woke up on June 17, 1998 to find that overnight you'd become too fat to consider yourself healthy, due to revised government definitions of "overweight."

Any "epidemic" can be increased when you change the rules midway. When the National Institutes of Health lowered the point at which people are defined medically as "overweight" they increased to 55% the number of Americans who will now be at risk for weight discrimination in employment and health insurance access. The market for weight loss treatment was also greatly increased, fueled by dire warnings in every "epidemic" announcement about rising health care costs associated with diabetes, hypertension and heart disease. But research shows these conditions can all be improved directly through lifestyle changes, independent of weight loss. This is all occurring, by the way, at a time in history when Americans are living longer than ever. And as Dr. Susan Wooley has sagely noted: "Even if people theoretically need it more, it doesn't make the weight loss treatments we have any more effective long-term."

The new NIH weight guidelines also tell doctors to advise "overweight" patients to lose weight at every medical visit. The NIH ignored the fact that fat people are already barraged with unsolicited weight loss advice when they go for medical, mental health and even vision and dental care. One research study found that embarrassment about weight and wanting to avoid another weight loss lecture was a major factor in female healthcare professionals' avoiding medical visits. Another study of almost 7000 women found that as weight increases, women are more likely to delay going in for pelvic exams, Pap smears and clinical breast exams. The researchers commented that this delay in care might account for some of the health risks attributed to weight alone. Well, finally! Large women and size acceptance advocates have been saying that for years.

Until every woman in the country can walk into health care settings that are free of weight bias, we won't be able to determine the extent to which delay of care, or inappropriate care, affects health outcomes. The WomanCare Plus project is a study Pat is working on with researchers from U.C. Berkeley's Center for Weight and Health. Data gathered from focus groups and surveys with both large women and healthcare providers will be used to eventually design better education programs for both groups. Debby's work, especially with her Body Positive Program, is promoting weight neutrality, a concept free of the bias so common in both medical and mental health care. She reminds us all: Assume nothing about behavior by looking at body size. As a health professional, until you assess and listen with compassion to the particular individual in front of you, you can't hope to help.

Finally, it is still heartbreakingly difficult to be a fat child. Teasing and torment surround them. Parents and schools must look at the extent to which this toxic environment impairs their learning and their health. Yet even simple changes could make a difference. Why, for instance, can't clothing manufacturers popular with kids and teens just add large sizes to what they already make and mix them right in with the other sizes? Not having to go to the "chub club" would be a very big deal to big kids. But weight prejudice undermines the health of all children, including those who are not fat. Girls as young as five are talking about their "fat thighs," and a study at Penn State found that at that tender age they already know about dieting. Dieting is as common in young people as listening to music—60-70% of teenage girls have dieted—and eating disorders plague youth of every ethnic and economic group. The journal *Pediatrics* recently reported that 9-13-year-olds consider smoking a way they might be able to lose weight.

While the NIH and most medical journals consistently focus on America's weight gain, and ignore these other issues, an unprecedented editorial appeared in the January 1, 1998 edition of the prestigious *New England Journal of Medicine*. Drs. Marcia Angell and Jerome Kassirer wrote "Losing Weight: An Ill-Fated New Year's Resolution" which is worth reading in its entirety. Here is the core message:

> Since many people cannot lose much weight no matter how hard they try, and promptly regain whatever they do lose...the $30-50 billion [spent] yearly, is wasted...Given the enormous social pressure to lose weight, one might suppose there is clear and overwhelming evidence of the risks of obesity and the benefits of weight loss. Unfortunately, the data linking overweight and death, as well as data showing the beneficial effects of weight loss, are limited, fragmentary and often ambiguous...Countless numbers of our daughters, and increasingly many of our sons, are suffering immeasurable torment in fruitless weight-loss schemes and scams, and some are losing their lives...Until

> we have better data about the risks of being
> overweight and the benefits and risks of trying
> to lose weight, we should remember that the
> cure for obesity may be worse than the condi-
> tion...Doctors should do their part to end
> discrimination against overweight people.

Bravo! We couldn't have said it better ourselves. We hope that as increasing numbers of health professionals and consumers get fed up with repeating the same old mistakes, that the Health at Every Size approach will become more commonplace.

New Resources

Great Shape is perhaps a women's history book, as much as it is a fitness and health book (check those 80's hairdos!!). There have been visible and welcome increases in the participation of women in sports since we first wrote of these issues—the victorious U.S. women's soccer team making the covers of *Time, Sports Illustrated, Newsweek and People Magazine* is but one example. But barriers to women's activity persist. With a booming economy and even more women working, lack of time for family, friends and necessary chores, let alone physical activity, remains a huge problem. But we still urge you to find as many of those ten minute breaks in your day as you can to enjoy moving and playing.

We are happy to say that clothing and exercise equipment to fit larger bodies is now much more available. You'll find lots of clothing stores and catalogues, as well as a variety of positive articles and other resources in magazines like *Radiance, BBW, Belle, and Mode.* Some of us have even had to learn to 'just say no' to yet another great colored t-shirt. Along with more clothing options, there is also increased acknowledgment in the fitness industry that 'hard bodies' are a turn-off to lots of people starting activity, not just those of us with 'soft bodies.' But there is a long way to go. One place where instructors and members of all sizes can relax and enjoy activity— without seeing scales, tape measures or diet products—is the Women of Substance Health Spa in Redwood City, California, whose owners Dana Schuster and Lisa Tealer were among the first Great Shape instructors. Even hard body clubs like World Gym in San Francisco can be accessible to large women when people like personal trainer Cinder Ernst create size-friendly classes and services. We hear of efforts like this all over the country. So, it's a new world out there, folks. Look for such programs and people in your area, and if you come up short you can at least find some support in cyberspace.

The Internet explosion is the biggest difference today in finding resources. Much of our Appendix is outdated, so check out the Web instead. If you don't have a computer, head to your local library or school. We've listed a few favorite web sites that will link you not only to us, but to the many wonderful people and places that support the ideas you'll read here. Some of our favorites:

Body Positive	http://www.bodypositive.com
Health at Any Size Web Ring	http://www.bodypositive.com/web_ring.htm
National Organization to Advance Fat Acceptance	http://www.naafa.org
Size Wise Search Engine	http://www.sizewise.com
Healthy Weight Network	http://www.healthyweight.net
Radiance Magazine	http://www.radiancemagazine.com
Junonia	http://www.junonia.com
BBW Magazine	http://www.bbwmagazine.com
Fat!So?	http://www.fatso.com
Vitality, Inc. (diet industry watchdog)	http://www.tiac.net/users/vtlty
New Paradigm Info for Health Professionals	http://msu.edu/user/burkejoy
Women of Substance Health Spa	http://www.women-of-substance.com
Cinder Ernst	http://www.cinderernst.com
Kelly Bliss	http://www.kellybliss.com
Melpomene Institute	http://www.melpomene.org
Fat Acceptance mailing list	majordomo@world.std.com SUBSCRIBE FAT-ACCEPTANCE-DIGEST
Fat and Fit mailing list	listproc@listserv.oit.unc.edu: SUBSCRIBE FATANDFIT [Your email address]

So, dear readers, we hope you enjoy *Great Shape* in its original form. We'll write other books in the future, perhaps. And we may see you in our travels around the country. But even if we never meet, rest assured that we think of you often with joy in our hearts. Be active. Be well. Be happy.

Pat Lyons
DebbyBurgard
January, 2000

Introduction

A book on exercise for large women?

An exercise book with pictures of women with flesh on their bones?

A book that says you can be active without waiting until you're size 7?

What sort of heresy is this?

We hope you are curious. We are a couple of rabble-rousers who want to open your mind to the idea that you have a right to play. This book is about the joy of moving in many different forms, from sports to dance. And while we think that everybody could use more of a playout than a workout in their lives, we are particularly fond of speaking out for large women.

We have watched ourselves struggle with the fitness culture. How many times have we started a diet, joined a health club, made a food chart, bought a protein supplement? How many times have we "blown" that diet, dropped out of the exercise class, and let the food chart and the unused cans of powder gather dust on the shelf? How many times can we put ourselves through that cycle of optimism, fatigue, and despair? We can answer that last question for ourselves: We will not go through it anymore. We got tired of it a long time ago, and we began to wonder: Why does this effort, which everyone assumes should work, so inevitably fail?

The answer is not simple. Some people say it's lack of will-power. But that doesn't fit with the evidence of our lives, which have been full of accomplishments, hard decisions, and commitments we have kept.

We decided to take a closer look at the whole cycle from start to finish in our own lives and in those of our friends. For most of us, no matter what our size, the motivation to exercise starts with the desire to lose weight. So we summon our courage and try a class—and walk away in a state of shock about how bad it felt, how painful the exercises were, how rushed the pace, and how embarrassing the experience of being the fattest person in the room. But as we limp away, we half think we *deserve* such a dismal experience for the sin of being fat. So we have doubts about challenging the instructor or the exercise club to serve us better. Instead, we just quietly drop out of sight. It relieves the pain of being in the class but leaves a residue of failure. We are unlikely to try *that* again!

It is time to pay attention to what does not work. The fitness industry, which tells us we are loathsome and lazy but maybe if we work real hard and punish ourselves they'll let us in the club, does not work. Gritting our teeth, holding our breath, and going for the burn does not work. Sweating it out for some future image of ourselves as a size 7 does not work.

So what works? Again, the answer is not simple. If by "what works" we mean "what helps people lose weight permanently," no one has come up with a satisfying answer. People can and do lose weight, but they tend to put it back on. Exercise does make bodies leaner, but it's not very dramatic. The process is slow, the results are not the stuff of "before" and "after" pictures, and they last only as long as you keep exercising.

What other purpose could there be to exercising?

We have found that some of the miseries we attributed to our weight were in fact miseries of lives without movement, lives without play, lives without deep breathing and zest. And lo and behold, movement, play, deep breathing, and zest could be ours *right now!*

Could physical activity be an end in itself?

That is the question we would like to pose to you, the question we invite you to explore.

An exercise book that is especially for large women?

This book is written for large women and anyone else who would like to understand the issues facing large women trying to be more physically active. We regard this book as only a beginning; while we have brought together as much information as we can, it is important to note that there are many areas where our knowledge is incomplete. We are not physicians, exercise physiologists, nutritionists, or any other kind of expert. We are two women who love physical activity. And because large women come in different sizes, with different needs, values, and experiences, this book cannot possibly be "complete." The world treats those who are 180 pounds differently from those who are 280 or 380 pounds. There are many books on this general subject yet to be written—for exercise leaders gearing their activities to larger bodies; for physicians caring for heavier athletes; for fat men, children, older people; and so on. There is much research yet to be done on why people maintain different body sizes; on the health effects of size discrimination; on the best ways to help people integrate movement into their lives; and so forth. We would like to open the exploration with this book.

You may have noticed that we have used the words *large* and *fat* in our discussion. Because there is such abhorrence of fat in our culture, the words to describe it are very controversial. The medical profession uses *obese,* but few fat people feel comfortable with that label, invoking as it does the image of a professional describing the disease of a patient. *Overweight* is commonly used by people trying to be polite, but it implies that there is an ideal lower weight to which fat people should conform. We believe that until the question is answered as to whether it is possible to maintain "ideal" weight permanently, it is misleading to use the term "overweight" (which is why it appears in quotation marks in this book). Until we understand the physiological processes underlying the maintenance of body size, using the term "overweight" just raises the question, "Over *what* weight?" With the new research on the genetic contribution to body size, it may be that in the future the term "overweight" will apply to people who are above their genetic weight, whatever size that is, rather than the "ideal" weight charts.

And so we come to *fat,* a word that has been used cruelly in our culture. In this book our use of the word *fat* is an attempt to normalize its meaning, to detoxify the word by using it in a matter-of-fact, descriptive way. There is no simpler, more apt word to describe fat than *fat.* But until people get used to hearing it in a matter-of-fact way, it will doubtless evoke painful associations. That is why we also use the term *large,* even though it is less precise. We are in a time of transition where our attitudes about and understanding of fat are undergoing changes. Perhaps the day will come when *large* will sound unnecessarily euphemistic, when *fat* will be heard in the same spirit as tall. But until then we want you to hear our message in spite of the awkwardness of our words.

An exercise book that has both sports and dance?

We are including a wide range of activities in this book. Why? Pat loves sports. I dance. Apparently the exercise preferences of large women are as varied as our tastes in books, movies, and vacation spots. There is no one activity that appeals to all large women any more than there is one activity that appeals to all thin women or hairy men or people with brown eyes!

The sports world traditionally has been male territory. Pat has worked toward women having equal access to that world. Her experience growing up in the Midwest in the fifties and sixties was very different from mine growing up in the Midwest in the sixties and seventies. Soccer, basketball, track and field events, and more, were off-limits to her but were routine gym classes to me because of the efforts of sporting women tired of traditional limitations. What was missing for me, though, was music and self-expression. And I have found that in dance. As you might guess, Pat has written the chapters about sports while I have written on aerobic dance and fitness. Our collaboration has made us aware of how split the two worlds usually are: Pat, in true jock style, wouldn't be caught dead in a leotard while I'll take up swimming in earnest when they invent an underwater Walkman. Give Pat running shoes and a finish line; give me leotards and a funky bass line! But give us both the bottom line of sharing our passions for movement with people who have been wrongly relegated to the sidelines.

Since this is an introduction, we would like to introduce ourselves.

Debby: I've loved to dance ever since I first sneaked downstairs, crashed my parents' parties, and found they couldn't bring themselves to send me back to bed as long as I boogied. Being a fiercely independent child, I scorned lessons as somehow cheating; the achievement was in teaching myself. Part of my fierce independence was an unwillingness to put myself in the position of being teased for being a stocky, early developing girl. But even at my highest weight (two hundred pounds in high school), I still danced at parties and watched "Soul Train," learning the pony, the mashed potato, the hustle, and so on. Finally, during my last year of college, I broke down and tried dance classes and found they weren't so bad.

After graduation I started studying traditional West African dance, and I found the drums, the rhythms, the sheer exuberance, intoxicating. A couple of my teachers were large women, and I remember the day one of them shook and shimmied her abundant hips and thighs in a fast, precise demonstration step past her transfixed students. I knew in my heart that I could never look like her because even though my butt was bountiful, it just wasn't bountiful enough. Oh, the drama of her shimmy! It was the first time I found myself envying a woman who was bigger than I was, and it was a revolutionary experience. It made me realize that our culture's current obsession with thinness is arbitrary; that in other places or in other times heavier bodies are or were seen as desirable; and that just as surely as thin bodies can be elegant and sleek, large bodies can have a different kind of dramatic and regal beauty.

While I was studying West African dance I began working with women (of all sizes) with eating disorders and body image disturbances. Our groups always benefited from the expertise of a movement therapist. She took people who would have preferred to stay numb below the chin and awakened them to their bodies. We did a lot of talking in those groups, and people found insight, but it seemed to me that movement therapy was always the moment of truth for group members who were so good at talking and so lost when it came to their bodies.

When I went west to go to graduate school for clinical psychology, I found an exercise class for large women in San Francisco called Fat and Fit. I had been so intrigued by the power of movement in African dance and in therapy groups, my response was, "It's about time!" No one was teaching such a class on the other side of the Bay, so I began We Dance. Pat and I first met one night when I substituted for Fat and Fit's instructor Eliza Mimski. Pat was talking with Eliza and her students in connection with her master's thesis research. Our paths kept crossing, and when the opportunity arose to co-write this book, we realized that her sports background and my dance background would challenge each of us to expand our notions of women's physical potential. Pat's intention to reclaim the traditionally male world of sports and my intention to reclaim the traditionally thin world of aerobic dance combined into a new model of physical activity: Recess for Grown-ups. It has been delightful!

Pat: I've always felt being able to play sports was a special gift, a potential I'd been given when the genetic cards were dealt. I was dealt a fat card, but I was also dealt this sporting ability and had the good fortune to grow up in a family that encouraged me to develop my potential. My mother made sure I took the free lessons offered by the recreation department and encouraged me to follow my interests while growing up. I was one of those kids who could always tell what season it was by the sports we were playing. In the summer we had swimming, bicycling, tennis, and the wonders of Girl Scout camp; in the winter we sledded like maniacs, and Mom transformed our backyard into a skating rink. My parents waltzed and jitterbugged their way through the years, never missed a Saturday night dance in all my formative years, and even paid for my brother and me to have Arthur Murray lessons. My mother is still an inspiration to me, since at seventy-three she still dances several times a week. I'm very thankful that sports and dancing were as much a part of our family as breathing.

I quit being active at about fifteen when I became more and more self-conscious about being fat. Physical education class was restricted to doing boring calisthenics indoors. Most of the girls were more worried about mussing their hairdos and getting out of taking showers than in lobbying for the same outdoor sports the boys had. Watching boys' football and basketball games became my replacement for the sweaty fun of my childhood activities. It was about then that I started dieting in earnest and began living "from the chin up" as a defense against all the negative carping about my being fat. If I'd kept playing, perhaps I would not have become so alienated from my body.

I spent my twenties dieting, smoking cigarettes, drinking, and surviving bouts of depression. Until I was thirty most of my sports experiences occurred during a few years of intense downhill skiing when I was twenty-four and twenty-five; mostly I watched sports on TV (usually with the guys, since most of my female friends weren't interested). Finally, urged on by a friend who helped me see that playing sports was much healthier than merely watching, I went back outside to play. I still love to watch sports, but now I try to spend just as much time playing.

During my thirties I devoted a great deal of time and energy to becoming healthy by playing tennis and softball, and going skiing, running, hiking, ice skating, and backpacking. While I didn't become magically thin, I surpassed my wildest dreams by running in a race I'd watched from the sidelines for years, backpacking to high mountain places, and ice skating by the light of the full moon on a frozen pond near my house. I found I loved physical activity for the ability it gave me to do something challenging and wonderful spontaneously. I had one cosmic experience after another in the great outdoors. All these physical memories are still stored in my body and have in fact replaced the pain buried there for so long, and I can recall them in a flash for inspiration.

I became healthier not only by becoming more physically active but also by learning to integrate my mind, spirit, and emotions into activity. I felt whole and wanted to find ways to share with other women the healing process I'd gone through. So at thirty-nine years of age I entered graduate school to study sport psychology and women's health. I began graduate school with the thought that the sport psychology techniques which had worked so well for me could also help women without a sports background to become more active. As is often the case in education, what I ended up learning was far beyond my expectations.

One day two wheelchair athletes came to speak to our sport psychology class. One of the women, a former gymnast who was paralyzed from the waist down as a result of a car accident, happened to look right at me when she addressed the class as "you temporarily able-bodied" folks. A shiver passed through me. I knew instantly what she meant. Some close calls I'd experienced had thoroughly convinced me that physical ability could be snatched away in one swift crash of metal. Disability such as that doesn't go away, and these athletes were facing challenges much greater than figuring out how to work exercise into their schedule. It was apparent that sports were not just something they did for exercise but also something they did to enrich their lives. For them it was a vehicle of empowerment and transformation. I knew the same had been true for me as a fat woman. My belief that sport was a force for healing was strengthened a hundredfold.

I also realized the same day that just because I was able to run then did not mean I'd always have the ability, and if exercise was going to be a permanent part of my life, I'd have to find lots of ways to keep the exhilaration, fun, and spirit of sport uppermost in my mind. The more physically challenged one is, the more courage and determination it takes to be active. Therefore, the effort to expand the experience of sport and dance beyond mere "exercise" became the central force of my work and ultimately the spirit in which this book was written.

Three years after entering graduate school, where I spent more time writing about sports than playing, I am forty pounds heavier and have given up the love of my life, running. I am simply not as able-bodied as I was a few years ago, but this does not mean I have returned to the couch. Now I walk instead of run and have rekindled my childhood love of swimming. Life changes, physical ability changes, but my love of movement has not changed. I love the feeling of suiting up in my running shoes and sweats, the idea of devoting playtime just to me, and the adventure of going out into the day curious about what enjoyment I'll find. I like to feel my muscles work and the heat build in my body, and I love the moments when my moving over the earth blends just right with the wind. I am more at peace with my body than I've ever been and know in my heart that if humans could fly I'd be out there trying. At the same time I know that humans can't fly; that, yes, I am temporarily able-bodied. But I also know that I can make the most of my ability, enjoy myself and be healthy, and no amount of poundage can stop me.

Overview of the Book

We would like to give you a sense of the scope and direction of this book. The first chapter, Fat *and* Fit, introduces the basic idea that you can have, and indeed deserve, physical activity in your life right now. It outlines the progress that large women are making in claiming this simple human pleasure for ourselves.

In Chapter 2 we try to give you some tools for assessing your own preferences in physical activity. What entices you? What has stymied your past attempts? We believe that becoming aware of all your feelings, not just the "motivational" ones, is the only way for you to learn to enjoy and feel safe venturing into this territory.

Once you have looked inside and determined your own unique preferences, you will find in Chapter 3 an explanation of the controversial and often confusing research on weight and exercise. What are you likely to achieve if you exercise, and what is unrealistic to expect? We also explain what makes exercise aerobic or not, and how to know if you are getting aerobic exercise. We get down to the very practical aspects of getting started. Where do you find clothes? How do you survive the health examination? What do you need to understand about the different sensations your body will experience during exercise?

Chapter 4 is the first chapter on physical activity itself, and we begin with warming up and stretching. No matter what activity you choose, warming up, stretching, and cooling down need to be a part of it. How are warm-ups different from stretches? When in your workout should you use these movements? After you've learned how to warm up and stretch, you can choose any of the activities highlighted in the following chapters as your activity.

For those of you interested in exercise and aerobic dance, Chapter 5 covers the We Dance program. The exercises are designed to strengthen common vulnerable areas such as the abdominal muscles (helping to support the lower back) and the knees and legs. We have also included a few of the dance steps from a typical We Dance class.

In Chapter 6 we cover walking, hiking, running, and swimming. Walking and swimming are the two activities most available to everyone; they are among the safest to do and can introduce you to the quiet pleasures of movement. We also explore hiking and running for recreation, and include ideas about organizing a group for your activity.

Chapter 7 covers information on sports. We acquaint you with a brief history of women in sports and an overview of possible activities you might like to try. We encourage you to let your ideas of possible activities range beyond what traditionally has been available to women, large or small.

Chapter 8 gives tips from the field of sport psychology to enhance your performance and enjoyment of any activity.

Finally, we include in Chapter 9 the inevitable ups and downs of making a change such as this in your life. We discuss the many barriers to large women exercising and how you can try to maintain your commitment to yourself in the face of pain, disappointment, and fatigue. We talk about how expecting to have those occasional downs can sometimes make it easier to get through to the other side because you know that "this, too, shall pass." Change is only smooth and straightforward in our fantasies, and we urge you to honor the uniqueness of your own path and keep traveling on it.

The appendices include many of the resources (books, clothes, classes, organizations, videos) we are aware of at this time. Our fervent hope is that by the time you read the list it will be incomplete because of all the new books, clothes, classes, organizations, and videos that will come out after our book!

The most difficult stage of the journey to a more active life is often the first twenty steps that get us out the door. This book is aimed particularly at helping you take these first steps. Now that we have introduced ourselves and our mission, we would like to plant an image in your mind as you begin this journey. It must be an image unique to you. Maybe it's an image you can recall, or maybe it's one you can paint afresh. Take yourself back to childhood: See yourself racing your best friend to the bus stop or playing tag after supper in the twilight or jumping rope double-dutch with the girls next door or playing foursquare until you dropped in a sweaty little heap. In short, picture yourself engaged in any kind of pleasurable physical activity. This, too, is exercise—this is recess!

And that is what this book is all about: putting the *play* back into a *workout.* This book is for you if you:

◆ have been turned off by the standard approach to exercise
◆ have felt afraid to become more active, worrying that you'd be hurt, embarrassed, or humiliated

- have tried being more active but dropped out because you became bored or burned out
- are involved in one activity and want to branch out to others
- are looking for respect as a large woman living in a size 7 world
- are simply looking for more fun in your life

If you've been longing to get a move on or have been wondering what it would feel like to be in great shape, now is the time to begin.

GREAT SHAPE

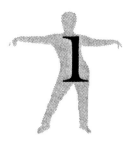

Fat and Fit

An Idea Whose Time Has Come

Envision a room filled with happy, healthy, dancing women. They twirl and swirl, stretch with catlike grace, and then . . . they get down, honey, and boogie to the beat. Sometimes they dance in a circle, laughing and playing a follow-the-leader game. They revive dances from the fifties and sixties—the stroll, pony, boogaloo, mashed potatoes—and make up steps of their own. After dancing themselves into a drenching sweat of pleasure, they cool down, slow down, relax, feel the flush in their cheeks, and luxuriate in the warmth of their bodies. This feels go-o-o-od deep down.

Now envision that all these healthy women weigh over two hundred pounds. Ooops. Did your mental TV screen short-circuit? Fat *and* fit? Did you find yourself mouthing the words *impossible, ridiculous?* Or did you say, "Hot damn, it's about time!"

The pleasures, benefits, challenges, and full-out exuberant fun of dance, sport, and movement are the birthrights of all people, not just the already athletic and fit. But larger women have been treated shabbily by the exercise establishment. Regardless of any polite veneer, the fat-hating attitudes of most instructors would make even the most stalwart believer in self-esteem cringe under their judgment. And it is very difficult to separate their hatred of the substance fat from their feelings toward you, a fat person. By not creating activities and environments that welcome us as we are, exercise enthusiasts who mistakenly equate *thinness* with *fitness* have made the *25 million women in America who are larger than a size 16* into objects of scorn. The standard exercise approach is either downright hostile to us, constantly exhorting us to lose our "ugly flab," or ignores our needs completely with blithe advice to "go at your own pace." It's no fun to be always out in right field or in the back row barely able to see an instructor and thus hopelessly out of step or driving yourself mercilessly to show them "fat women can do it."

There is a seemingly universal assumption that we are fat because we refuse to adhere to the engraved-in-stone moral code of "eat less and exercise more." Because we've been "bad," it is further assumed that we deserve to be the butt of jokes and the bad examples held up to other women lest they "let themselves go" and end up looking like us. It seems most exercise devotees have to assume this stance because the pursuit of a fat-free body forms the underlying motivation for their participation in physical activity.

We believe in participation for its own sake, for the sheer pleasure of it. We further believe that it is the existence of prejudice and discrimination toward fat people that most severely undermines our well-being, and very often it is precisely what keeps many of us from becoming more physically active—hence more healthy—in the first place. And we think it's time to stop allowing ourselves to be victimized by such attitudes. If we can't change society's attitudes, we can at least change our own.

Not content to sit on the sidelines and tired of the social and physical put-downs, to say nothing of the very real risks of exercise geared for thin folks, large women have formed our own activities paced for bigger bodies: swims, hikes, belly dance classes, canoe and cross-country ski trips, dance and aerobics classes. A trapeze act in the San Francisco Bay Area called Fat Chance provided the groundwork for these activities a few years ago by demolishing stereotypes about what strong, fit, fat women could do. The message is clear: We do not have to be ashamed of our fat. We have a right to move and groove and sweat and strain and have fun and love ourselves as we are. And no one but no one need give us any grief about our size.

Physically active large women have found that we can be fat *and* fit. We don't have to wait for a size 7 body to have efficient hearts, capable and graceful bodies, and good feelings about our physical selves. Many of us have reversed our collective "couch potato" self-images. We've discovered that our bodies, like all human bodies, hunger to move; our muscles, too, itch to be used; our spirits yearn to play. If you think of yourself as totally sedentary and can't imagine wanting to move, stop and ask yourself how you felt the last time you had to ride in a car for eight hours or stand in line at the bank for an hour? That cramped, antsy feeling is your body saying, *"Move!"* And we all have it, this pressing need for movement, no matter our size, no matter how long it has been since we've been active.

We deserve the self-confidence and pleasure of having responsive, capable bodies. All day, every day, virtually all women internalize the overwhelming media message that "thin is best"—driven home by commercials with gorgeous, leotard-clad models dripping sweat into their diet drinks—and we feed ourselves a litany of self-degrading thoughts: If I was thin like her, my life would be perfect. I hate my thighs, my stomach, my upper arms; maybe my ankles are okay, and I have a nice smile. If I'd just stick to a diet I'd be able to fit into that new dress that's still too small, and so on, ad nauseum, ad oblivion, ad insanity! What are we waiting for!

Many of us have finally come to the conclusion that picking a number on the scale and postponing our lives until we reach that number is never going to work. What we really want is a good life, full of friends, enjoyment, and self-respect. To eat what we want when we feel hungry, stop when we're full, move when we feel sluggish, tense, or in need of a lift or some fun, and stop when we're refreshed—and *then* see what our body size is and make peace with it—is, quite simply, a way of living that feels good. And we can have it—now and forever. It is a good life that is *possible.*

So if you're not out there giving yourself this good life, we hope that this book will show you what you're missing and nudge you on your way. With as much solid information, support, and inspiration as we can pour into these pages, we're asking you to stretch both your body and your image of yourself and your possibilities. We're not saying it'll be easy, necessarily, but if you've been agonizing about your weight, then your life until now has probably not been easy either. We *are* saying it can be fun to learn, to grow, to discover. And make no mistake about this, it certainly is about time. For all of us!

A Racy Story

Before the race I was nervous, feeling as though I'd swallowed a dozen butterflies that were now running their own race round and

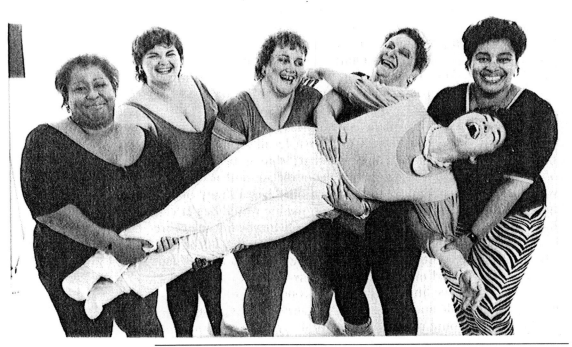

We Dancers Peggy Wilson, Frances White, Carol Squires, Robin Hopkins, Rosemary Senegal, and a reclining Debby Burgard.

round in my stomach. I'd never run a race before, let alone one with fifty thousand people, but I had my heart set on finishing–not winning, mind you, but simply running the whole way. A friend said I could walk for a while if I got tired, but I knew it wouldn't be the same. I'd trained for months for this once impossible dream, and here it was stretched out in front of me. All I had to do now was do it. The roar of the crowd signaled the start of the race, and off we went. Running, I was now too busy to worry about the butter-flies.

The Bay to Breakers racecourse covers 7.6 miles of the city of San Francisco, from the edge of the Bay on the city's east side to the breakers at the ocean. An annual event that started in the early 1900s with a few stalwart "kooks," it turned into a costumed, moving block party for thousands during the fitness boom of the seventies. I used to walk down to the bottom of my street every year and sit and smoke cigarettes while the runners whizzed by, wondering what it would take for me to be able to move with such ease. Now, a few years later, here I was, number 17,291 on my chest, facing my biggest physical challenge ever. How different I was feeling on this gloriously sunny Sunday than on years of Sundays past.

When I started running at age thirty-three I was a five-foot eight-inch, 190-pound, two-pack-a-day smoker with a scary cough. I played tennis fairly regularly but could only run a block at a time nonstop. Every day I'd run a block, go home, smoke a cigarette, and congratulate myself that I'd been out there trying. After about a month I was running two to three blocks and smoking fewer cigarettes. I started reading everything I could get my hands on about aerobic exercise, women's sports, feminism, sport psychology, nutrition, and wellness, and finally came to believe that I could actually make a difference in my health. Although I'd been a nurse for many years, I knew mostly about illness and medical treatment; I didn't actually know much about becoming or staying healthy. I began really learning about health by trying to become healthy myself, and running seemed like the most direct route to improvement. I figured I'd lose weight, too, if only I could run far enough or fast enough. About the third month of running I quit my twenty-year smoking habit, something I'd tried unsuccessfully to do on several previous occasions. What a reward! Still, it took a year before I could run a mile. In another year I was able to run three miles and began fantasizing about running the Bay to Breakers. Could it be possible? The next thing I knew it was Bay to Breakers Sunday, and I was facing the Hayes Street hill.

The Hayes Street hill (Heartbreak Hill, as some rather melodramatically inclined folks dubbed it years ago) is a sharp contrast to the flat plains of downtown San Francisco, and it was this hill I feared, only two miles into the racecourse. If I had to walk there, it might be too hard to start running again. I concentrated on my breathing—in . . . out . . . in . . . out—and started up the hill. Drawn upward by the hup, hup, hup chant of the crowd and hypnotized by the thousands before me whose heads all appeared to be bouncing in unison with the hup, hup beat, the hill slowed me down some, but I kept running.

The first block passed, no problem. Hey, this isn't so bad. By the second block I could hear a band at the top of the hill five blocks away playing the theme song from *Rocky,* a movie about going the distance. A little shot of inspiration. The second block passed more quickly than the first. Now it seemed that rather than slowing down, the crowd decided to go faster up the hill, rising to the challenge. The third block whizzed by, and I felt a giggle rise in my throat. I was going to do it, I could tell! By the time I finally got to the top of the hill I was laughing and ready to dance in a circle. The supposed heartbreak of Hayes Street hill was instead a piece of cake! It was all downhill to the ocean from there.

Rounding the corner onto Divisadero Street, I was still a bit giddy from my uphill run. I slapped hands with one rather grizzled character on the sidelines who was exhorting runners to "gimme five," and in that second we celebrated my determination. "Thataway, sister, all the way to the ocean," he said with a wink as I ran on.

The last four miles of the course ran through Golden Gate Park, the scenic route for sure, past the beds of flowers at the conservatory, the magical rhododendron garden, and some very bored buffaloes. At about mile five I began to tire. I had already run farther than ever before, and my legs were complaining loudly. Thank goodness for the costumed crazies around me—people dressed as bowling balls, a six pack of beer, a gorilla, Santa Claus, and a few free spirits who wore nothing at all. I let my attention focus on all the silliness to ignore my aches and pains, and I remembered this last two-mile stretch was a gentle downhill coast to the finish. I could see the ocean vividly in my mind because I'd trained with this image, planting it firmly in place. Between concentrating on my ocean image and the gorilla in front of me, I kept up my pace.

In training for the race I'd also made it a practice to run "just a little farther" even at the point when I felt I could run no more. Sometimes it was only a few steps; other times it was another mile or so. If I wasn't feeling any true pain but was simply tired, I made this into my signal to stretch myself, to try for just a bit more. Luckily I was able to snatch this little psychological boost out of my bag of tricks just when I needed it most, during that last mile. I could hear the roar of the crowd at the finish line, and watchers along the route encouraged us with applause and advice to "hang in there, you're almost through."

I was tired, with legs aching and running really slowly, one foot in front of the other, when finally the finish line appeared ahead. Cheering bystanders formed a long tunnel to run through, so in one last burst of energy and bravado I sprinted the last one hundred yards. I crossed the finish line with a rush of excitement, exhilaration, accomplishment, pride, and sheer happiness that I'd never felt before. This satisfaction must be what champion athletes feel, along with being absolutely crazy with delight. I put on my souvenir T-shirt and wore it as if it were my very own Olympic gold medal.

I finished the 7.6-mile course in one hour forty-five minutes. There are those who say "real" runners go much faster than that, but what did I care? I wasn't even supposed to be able to run. I was labeled *obese* by medical types, and three months after I'd started running I read in a fitness book that people more than thirty pounds "overweight" shouldn't run, that they should lose weight before running. Fortunately I read that *after* I'd discovered the challenge, exuberance, and rewards of running, or I might never have had the Bay to Breakers to celebrate. I was fat but I was fit, and no one could take that away from me.

My health had improved dramatically since my first days of running. My resting pulse went from one hundred to sixty; my blood pressure, while always normal, lowered slightly; seemingly endless bouts of depression, that I'd experienced for years, lifted; my cigarette-related colds became virtually nonexistent; and my flexibility, strength, and lung power improved enough to play softball at the third base position and to backpack to over ten thousand feet. I threw away my scale and stopped dieting once and for all and concentrated on eating whole, nutritious foods. All things considered I was much healthier at age thirty-five than I was at twenty-five, the year I weighed 139 after a crash dieting spree. But despite all these positive changes and being at the peak of my activity level, running, skiing, playing softball, and backpacking, I never attained my "ideal" weight. I was in the best shape of my life but at 185 pounds and 35% body fat I had not become magically thin. The truth was apparent: I could be fit and healthy, but I'd always be fat.

I ran in three more Bay to Breakers over the next five years, the last time weighing 215. That last time, a woman a little larger than I was running very near me. We smiled at each other in a shy, almost secret, knowing way that acknowledged we were breaking the rules, flouting the stereotyped expectations people have of us. Fat people are lazy. Fat people hate to exercise. Fat people don't deserve respect. Fat people can't be healthy and fit. Oh yeah?

"If Only for Your Health, Dear . . ."

If we larger women had a nickel for every time we received unsolicited advice about weight and pooled those nickels together, we could buy Hawaii! Just think: permanent vacations on the beach of our choice . . . balmy nights on romantic verandas . . . exotic trips into lush tropical jungles . . . swimming in crystal clear lagoons with flowers in our hair.

There are few things more insulting than having a relative, friend or, amazingly enough, a total stranger hand you a diet book or article about weight loss, professing concern for your health as justification for rudeness. Sometimes they slip in the phrase, "You have such a pretty face . . ." allowing our imagination to infer how ugly they think our body is. They try to shame us into "caring about ourselves." In the words of eating disorders specialist Susan Wooley, "If shame could cure obesity, there wouldn't be a fat woman in the world."

NOW HEAR THIS—all relatives, friends, mates, children, co-workers, and especially total strangers—CEASE AND DESIST! You are not helping to make us healthier. You are part of the problem. We have tried more diets than you can believe and have only become fatter as a result. Please let *us* decide what is healthy and proceed from our own knowledge. Thank you. (This message has been brought to you by the Society for the Prevention of Cruelty to Women of Substance.)

There are people who will argue to the death that fat people cannot be healthy and fit, that the terms fat and fit are mutually exclusive. While experts will continue to disagree, even contradict one another on the actual health risks of fat, you need not wait for their consensus to become more fit and healthy regardless of your weight. Resigning yourself to the idea that "fat people can't be healthy" just because everyone says so can become a self-fulfilling prophecy. But that is unnecessary. There are definite things you can do to improve your health. Most important is to define what health means to you and reach for that goal.

You can educate yourself by reading what knowledgeable people have written, and we have included our own ideas as well as a multitude of other resources for you to check out. But remember the wisdom of not believing everything you read. The experts don't agree, and much of what has been written about fat and health, particularly the information found in diet books, is not only untrue but dangerous. We encourage *you* to become an expert on *your own body,* learn what works for you, and not rely on distant experts for "the truth."

After everything we have read, heard, discussed, and thought about, we have come to the conclusion that the scientific understanding of why people develop and maintain their body fat is primitive at best. There are at least twenty-five different ways to cause weight gain in laboratory animals and probably that many or more in humans. The standard advice to "eat less and exercise more" sounds simple enough, but if it actually worked, why would there be a new diet or fitness book published every twenty minutes? What else would there be to say? The implication is that it is we who are at fault—no willpower, you understand—rather than the methods that are being pushed, published, and proselytized, or even the goals themselves.

We can tell you for sure what doesn't work—dieting. Ninety-five to ninety-eight percent of people who lose weight by dieting gain it back and find it harder to diet the next time, and pay both a physical and an emotional price in the process. Yet try to find a magazine or newspaper without ads for some miracle diet product! The yo-yo cycle of dieting and inevitable weight regain is clearly not a healthy regimen for anyone. Even exercise, which can be a direct health enhancer, is not a miracle cure for losing fat. Most people will lose a moderate amount of fat when they become more active, but there is no proven way for fat people to lose large amounts of weight permanently.

Society's headlong pursuit of fat-free bodies, without regard to risk, cost, or lack of long-term success, has lead to the proliferation of both humiliating and health-threatening measures. Every morning for four months, after eating breakfast, a woman in Oregon who was trying to lose seventy-five pounds put on a plastic face mask custom-made with holes that would allow only a straw to reach her lips; she lost five pounds. Surgical techniques are the most extreme measures and are reserved for only the heaviest people because they entail significant risks. According to Dr. Paul Ernsberger, a post-doctoral biomedical research fellow at Cornell University, "Weight-loss surgery, including intestinal bypass operations, has probably already killed well over a hundred times as many people as toxic shock syndrome," but there have been no screaming headlines to bring this fact to light. With the prejudice and discrimination that fat people face, it is no surprise that out of desperation people will try almost anything to lose weight. There are even some who say they wouldn't mind dying if they could be thin at their funeral, which does seem rather extreme, particularly under the guise of weight loss as a health-enhancing measure.

Myths, Mysteries and Motivation: Defining Health for Yourself

Fat people are barraged by contradictory advice from all sides, some of it from "experts," some from friends, relatives, and even strangers, some from out-and-out crackpots—and none of it adds up to any kind of consensus. Depending on where we look we are told to diet, not to diet, to exercise, to lose weight before exercising, to forget about weight loss, and to lose weight or die early. In the midst of these confusing and conflicting messages we are above all supposed to motivate ourselves and get out there and *do something.* ANYTHING. The message we internalize is that we are not okay the way we are but must somehow create dramatic change. The fact that overnight dramatic change rarely lasts is lost in the shuffle. The words "trim and fit" roll off the tongue of every health and fitness educator so often that we come to equate weight loss with success and good health. And most Americans have been convinced that anything less than total success means shameful failure.

A vigorous and diligent participant in a jogging class described her elation after two years attending the class: "I feel great! My blood pressure came down so I don't have to take my medicine anymore, I'm full of more energy at fifty-three than ever before, and I just love to come to these classes because we have such a good time." Then she hung her head in obvious sadness, even shame. "I haven't lost any weight, though. I eat a good, nutritious diet and don't have any traces of high blood sugar anymore, but I still weigh about the same as when I started. I don't know what I'm doing wrong." How has our society's distorted view of success convinced this vigorous, enchanting human being that ultimately, despite all of the improvements she could see in her health, she had failed? That she should agonize one moment is a disgraceful example of how societal attitudes have undermined her self-respect.

How many of us have agonized about our bodies and experienced failure over and over again in the familiar arena of dieting when in reality dieting has only made us fatter and reinforced our sense of hopelessness? Defining weight loss as success and anything else as failure is certainly not conducive to developing positive self-esteem. And since we must have self-esteem to motivate ourselves to improve our health, it is obvious that we must redefine success. To do that we have to arm ourselves with accurate information and a strong will to challenge standard ideas about our potential for health and self-respect at whatever our weight is. This is where a positive definition of health begins.

All of this is not to say that we oppose weight loss. Many of you bought this book hoping to lose weight by becoming more active, and we are not foolish enough to pretend that reading our words will remove this desire. Our point is that some of you may lose a moderate amount of weight and others may not, but all of you can make improvements in your mental and physical well-being through the joys of physical movement. We are not invested in whether you lose weight or not. We do not consider weight loss a criterion of success. We *are* invested in your finding ways to become as healthy as you can be, and on your own terms. We are also invested in alleviating any sense of failure you may feel when weight loss does not occur in response to changes you make. If your body is meant to be fatter than what society says is okay in the 1980s, you can still learn to enjoy and value the body you have now—not the mythical one society says you could or should have.

Rather than obsessing about the quantity of food allowed on a "diet" or the minimum number of minutes you have to exercise for it to "do any good," you can start a new approach now: Look for ways to spend more time enjoying yourself. Nourish yourself with healthy food. Treat yourself to a massage on a regular basis. Find friends to exercise and play with, and join with others to fight prejudice and discrimination against fat people. It is much more fun to *add* positive changes to your life than to constantly look for what you think you must stop doing.

Given what large women have had to put up with, it is not surprising when some of us assert our right *not* to exercise. Remember that exercise is not a duty of fat people. We have no more obligation to exercise than anyone else. Consider our words as an invitation to be more active, not as another mandate from people you've never met. We believe that large women can and do enjoy exercise but only when we are treated, and treat ourselves, with respect. Physical activity is a way to nourish our bodies, not reduce them; a way to enrich our lives, not punish ourselves.

There is an erroneous idea that becoming more fit is like getting on an elevator on the ground floor and zooming up to the twenty-seventh floor, jumping out, and getting a fitness award for life. Not so. Just as life is a process of growth and change, so are changes in your health and level of fitness. The *process* can be your focus, not an anticipated end result. It is also important not to limit your definition of health only to "fitness." Physical fitness is but one aspect of a healthy person. While people capable of running marathons may be in great physical shape, they may be so competitive that they are lousy mates, parents, or bosses.

Becoming more healthy encompasses something beyond just physical fitness. It is the process of developing a balance and harmony among the physical, mental, emotional, spiritual, environmental, and social aspects of your life. And you cannot achieve this balance immediately. It takes time—days, months, and years. Relax. There is no emergency. You have the rest of your life to learn

behaviors that will enhance the quality of your life. The most important part of the entire process is to stop hating yourself because you
are "too fat." Hating yourself is a far greater obstacle to positive
health than any amount of fat on your body. Learning to accept your
body brings you one step closer to your goal of positive health.

As you become more active you may also notice another change
that has benefits of its own: a desire to learn more about nutrition.
As you learn to nourish yourself with exercise, you may find that you
also choose to nourish yourself with the vitamins, minerals, and
other energy boosters nutritious foods contain so you can keep
going. If you have ever lived in the malnourished state of dieting,
existing on diet drinks and food substitutes instead of *food,* then you
know how deprived and depressed it is possible to feel. You can also
become malnourished and feel lousy from eating food with lots of
chemical additives and preservatives, or with too much sugar, salt,
and fat, at the expense of more nutritious foods. The more you begin
to care about your body, the more you will begin to care about what
you put in it. Experimenting with changing the foods you eat is a
very gradual process, one that can go on for years. You will learn
what your body really wants for nourishment as you unlearn any
deprivation-ridden dieting behavior.

Dieting may initially feel like control—over your appetites and
thus your life—but almost inevitably it gives way to a binge, followed
quickly by shame over losing control. The punishing cycle of dieting
and bingeing, and the accompanying preoccupation with the size of
our bodies during every waking moment, is a modern-day form of
foot binding, and it can be as paralyzing emotionally as foot binding
was physically.

In a 1986 study of five hundred girls conducted by the University of California at San Francisco, nearly half of the nine-year-olds
and eighty percent of ten- and eleven-year-olds reported they were
already dieting, establishing this tragic cycle at an age when fun,
games, and kid adventures should be their main challenge. These are
our daughters and they deserve better. Sound nutrition, not dieting,
is the foundation of health for every child and every adult. Until we
learn to love ourselves and our bodies from the inside out, instead
of looking into mirrors to tell us if we are acceptable, we will not
have the freedom to pursue fulfilling lives. Until we learn what kind
of food we are truly hungry for and feed ourselves with love and care,
neither we nor our daughters will have the energy to become the
athletes and dancers we may have only dreamed about until now.
And how can any of us possibly enjoy recess if we're so busy counting
calories and judging ourselves!

A Call to Recess

Gales of hysterical laughter came billowing over the hill as I drove
up to the Radiance Retreat site. *Radiance: The Magazine for Large
Women,* published in Oakland, California, operates from a basic
premise of respect for women of all sizes of large. Entertaining and
informative articles on the arts, health, fashion, and the like, blend
with feature stories about large women enjoying fulfilling lives.
Without putting down thinner women, the magazine simply encourages women all sizes of large to stop putting their lives on hold
until they lose weight and to get on with the challenge and fun of
living life to its fullest. Publisher Alice Ansfield began sponsoring
retreats for her readers in 1985.

Since the very beginning these gatherings felt the way Girl
Scout camp used to—safe for me to be me and wildly fun. The
retreats are always held at some lush, remote place surrounded by
forests of beauty and silence, but unlike most Girl Scout camps, they
are blessed with amenities such as swimming pools, hot tubs, and
decidedly better meals. Everyday life, full of rules and petty insults,
can seem miles away as exploring the out-of-doors, playing with
friends, and learning new things become the main goals. These
retreats are the best form of recess for adults I've found because no
one is left out, and any pain experienced at the end of the weekend
is likely to be from sidesplitting laughter.

Every retreat has a speaker or focus—in fact, the philosophy of
"fat and fit," complete with aerobics and dance classes, was presented
at the first Radiance Retreat. Some women have taken their first hike
in years on these occasions, while others swim, read a good book,
or just relax in the sun. For some it's the first time they've ever been
with a large group of women, let alone a group of large women, and
this experience of sharing warmth, acceptance, support, and a feeling of belonging is inspiring.

There is always enough of a sense of security to allow for honest
conversations about our struggles as larger women. We share everything, from the pain and frustration of discrimination to where to
get good deals on large-size clothing or a bra that fits decently.
Coming together as "just us" and knowing no one is going to hassle
us about our size or whether we eat dessert makes it safe for us to
share all sides of ourselves and take some risks. Women who have
always felt ashamed of their bodies meet women who have overcome
both shame and shyness and enjoy nude sunbathing. Women who
have struggled with discrimination in the job market meet others
who will happily share their secrets of determination and success—as

lawyers, computer experts, counselors, managers, secretaries, writers, carpenters, teachers, nurses, business women, and dance and
fitness educators.

Because we face prejudice we must necessarily learn to deal with
pain and overcome obstacles. To do so we can learn from others but
must also learn to be ourselves—to be serious when life calls for it
but also to play, act silly, cackle hysterically, dance, sing, and be as
outgoing as we might be more often if perhaps we didn't fear the
insults that so frequently come our way. Most of all, these retreats
offer large women a way to overcome isolation, a killer disease, and
that alone leads to improved health.

Stop and think about the last time you saw a group of, say, six
women over two hundred pounds out in public together. It's pretty
rare, right? Fat people have learned that we are supposed to be
invisible (a contradiction in terms when you think about it), and
many of us actually try to become invisible by wearing dark clothes
or by staying home. In the words of swimmer, dancer, and NAAFA
(National Association to Advance Fat Acceptance) member Frances
White: "Isolation is the worst thing that happens to large people.
They're told that they are unattractive, ungainly, whatever. And they
buy it. They listen to it and withdraw from life. The most important
thing about Debby's We Dance class is that it brought us out of our
shells. It allows us to be physical in a safe forum, and it allows
improvement at our own speed, without feeling that we have to
compete against anybody else."

Rosemary Senegal, another avid Radiance retreater and We
Dance enthusiast, puts it this way:

> Outsiders tried to make me feel strange as a child because I was fat,
> but I knew a lot of love from my family. When I was a teenager, I
> lost some weight so that when I married I was wearing a size 16 dress.
> My husband had never liked fat women, but he married me for
> reasons more important than my size, but knowing I was going to
> get fatter because I told him I was going to get fatter! After I was
> married, I went from a size 16 to a 20. And I kind of withdrew. I'd
> go on and off diets, up and down, and felt bad about myself because
> I was not accepting myself and that was really tough.
>
> Then a friend of mine started going to dance class, and I said
> I'd go with her for a lark because she didn't want to go alone. And
> I rediscovered my love for dancing. As a teenager and young adult
> I danced all the time, and finding this class is probably one of the
> greatest things that happened to me in my adult life. Even my hus-
> band has started to change his mind about the way he feels about
> fat—he's one of those notoriously thin men who's never been over

140 pounds in his life—and it's real tough for him to understand where you are in being a big person. But just watching me come out of a shell I was in for a long time—both through my class and through Radiance—has helped him tremendously to understand.

Rosemary, Frances and the many other large women involved in Bay Area retreats and exercise groups have not only learned to come out of their shells but have made some lasting friends in the process.

Friends Are Good Medicine

"Make new friends but keep the old; one is silver and the other gold." Okay, all you former Girl Scouts, does that little refrain stir old memories? If it seems that you've always felt better after being with a close friend, you're not imagining things. It not only feels good to give and receive support from those around you, but it also does wonders for your health as well. In recent years medical scientists have documented the relationship of positive social support—networks composed of family, friends, neighbors, co-workers, and presumably other Girl Scouts—to improvements in both mental and physical health. The results of these studies, which initiated a statewide Friends Are Good Medicine campaign in California a few years ago, are fascinating:

A nine-year study of seven thousand residents of Alameda County, California, found that people with few relationships with other people had death rates *two to five times higher* than those with more ties. The differences were independent of all the usual health risk factors of smoking, drinking, lack of exercise, and of psychological variables or utilization of health services. This finding appeared for both sexes, for all ethnic groups, and across socioeconomic lines (Berkman/Syme, 1979).

A 1975 study investigated the levels of life stress and social support in women who had recently experienced a severe depression. The women who experienced severe life stress events and did not have a confidant, someone they could trust and talk with about their real feelings, were approximately *ten times* more likely to be depressed than women who did have a confidant. "A large number of superficial friendships seemed to be of little value in mediating depression; a close, intimate relationship was found to be the most important variable" (Brown, 1975).

The relationship of stress to the development of various illnesses has been discussed in serious medical literature and popular self-help books. What is not as well known is that people who experience life's stresses in isolation are at greater risk for problems.

Social prejudice against fat people, a source of great stress in itself, is so common that it is not surprising many of us end up in isolation. Even self-help groups, which operate from the assumption that it is easier to reach out to others who share a common experience, can be problematic when the common experience has a basis in social stigma, for the stigmatized may not wish to share one another's company. You may have no other fat friends, for instance, or might never consider dating a fat person. As fat women, we may have learned not only to hate ourselves but to hate others like us too. Even more common than hatred is distancing: We look at a woman fatter than ourselves and breathe a sigh of relief that we are "not as fat as she is." We distance ourselves from women larger than ourselves because we are overwhelmed by fear that we may become like them, and we staunchly refuse to acknowledge any similarities we may share. And this makes all of our lives more difficult than they would be if we were willing to reach out to one another.

To reach out to other large women and, even more unconventional, to do so outside the familiar context of searching for a "cure" for fat was the inspiration of a group of women calling themselves the Fat Underground in the early 1970s. It was these women who, by sharing the truth of their real lives, came to the conclusion that dieting not only doesn't work but is harmful, and that fat people don't eat more than thin people. It has taken the medical community years to even read, let alone believe, the scientific research that has been conducted to back up Fat Underground's vision. And there are still many who resist the facts, including a great number of fat people. To accept the fact of being fat forever can be very difficult (some people have compared it to accepting the idea of death) and can create panic and deep resistance. Rather than being consoled by the facts, you may instead hope against hope that all of the research on genetic causes of fat and the failure of diets is wrong. It is difficult to give up the idea of never being thin, and you may not feel like giving up this positive dream for yourself.

In the words of Ellyn Satter, nutritionist, psychotherapist, and author of *Child of Mine: Feeding with Love and Good Sense:* "The Cinderella myth has led many women to waste their lives waiting to become thin. My advice is live today as if you will be fat forever because in the real world there are few Cinderellas." Acceptance of yourself as a self-respecting fat woman eager to get on with your life is a process that will be gradual. But it's harder to do by yourself; it will help to share your struggle with others.

Women have come together in groups to bemoan their fat for years—just ask the millionaires of Weight Watchers—but to come together in nonjudgmental encouragement and curiosity, to share both accurate information and support, is another ball game entirely. It can be scary and exhilarating at the same time. It can also be incredibly empowering; it can give you the confidence to challenge and then begin to let go of any of your own anti-fat attitudes. The next step is to tackle these attitudes in the outside world.

If *we* are not interested in believing sound scientific research and in changing the fat-hating attitudes in the world that hurt us, then who will be? And while changing the world's attitude toward fat people from ridicule to respect may not be totally possible in our lifetime, it is certainly worth the effort to try, especially since it gets us together with others. Whether this is done in exercise classes, in special getaways such as Radiance Retreats or in any other context, the mere fact of joining with people like ourselves in something we believe in can be beneficial to our health by bringing us out of isolation. In his book, *Anatomy of an Illness,* Norman Cousins described watching Marx Brothers movies as therapy to heal a killer disease because laughter positively stimulates the body's immune system. Thus the combination of positive social support and laughter would seem to be an especially powerful booster for good health. So make way—large laughing women coming through!

The thing that was always best about recess was the fact that you could play with your friends, making up the rules as you went along, and the teachers mostly stayed out of the way. Radiance Retreats and other gatherings of large women will become more and more popular as large women realize we can still make up the rules as we go. Instead of just accepting the putdowns of a world that says get skinny or get lost, we can find our own games to play in if necessary. With respect both to recreational games and the game of life, we can decide for ourselves how we wish to play and can create situations for ourselves that maximize our pleasure and our health. When it comes to becoming more physically active there are plenty of large women in the world who are itching for a good time. Let's get together and do it!

Some of the Things that Could Stop You (But Won't)

The Couch-Potato Syndrome

If you think of yourself as a couch potato, look around—there are spuds of all sizes lounging right there with you. While some other societies dance through life as a matter of course, the American life-style is much more sedentary, emphasizing a service economy in the workplace and gadgets and convenience at home. The result is a powerful cultural barrier to activity. Where once fifty percent of American labor involved vigorous physical activity, it now is estimated that only two percent of American adults get adequate amounts of exercise for health in their jobs. A 1986 Department of Health and Human Services report estimated that only "ten to twenty percent of adult Americans engage in the kind of regular exercise most likely to ensure cardiovascular fitness." As a nation we spend our workday sitting—at desks, in cars, in classrooms—and spend much of our recreation time this way as well, watching sports or watching our children play rather than playing ourselves.

Our children are much less active now too, however. While in the fifties our mothers used to beg us to come in from playing outside when it was dark, mothers now have to beg their kids to turn off the television and go outside to play. It is estimated that the average American teenager will have spent more than twenty-two thousand hours in front of a television by the time she graduates from high school. As a nation we have become watchers, not doers, with the remote control TV switch the symbol of our transformation into couch potatoes.

Research by sport sociologist Susan Greendorfer and others shows that adult women who are active in sports received strong family encouragement when they were young and physical activity was a regular part of family interactions. While school plays an important role in encouraging sports participation for boys, this has not been found to be true for girls. In other words, if our daughters are going to be able to dance or belt a softball into the outfield, as parents we must encourage their early participation and not think the schools are taking care of that task for us.

Children who are not encouraged to dance or play physically demanding games and sports never adequately learn skills of physical coordination; their reflexes do not develop to their fullest capacity, and their confidence in their body's ability to bring them joy is not firmly established. If they are ridiculed for being fat or for any lack of innate ability, either by peers, teachers, or parents, they will carry this scar with them, making participation in adulthood even more difficult.

In childhood we are not only at our highest level of physical energy but also at our lowest level of physical fear, unless we have been taught to be afraid. Young children are not usually afraid of hurting or embarrassing themselves. They will repeat the same action dozens of times in order to get it right because they don't have adult inhibitions about making mistakes and because repetition is often just another word for playing. Children are open and ready to try new challenges because risks seem like no big deal.

As we get older, and particularly as adults, we become afraid of breaking a leg, splitting our pants, looking foolish or clumsy, or otherwise damaging our bodies or our dignity. Too often we then decide on the "safe" course of not trying at all. Therefore, the best favor you can do the children in your life is to intervene early in sedentary patterns and encourage them to experiment and challenge themselves in dance, sports, and games that help them learn to trust their bodies. Participating with them in physically active family outings will benefit everyone. And if they take physical education in school be sure that their teachers understand you expect them to treat your child with respect regardless of size or abilities.

There is nothing quite like a childhood memory of exhilaration and accomplishment to get an adult off the couch and back into the world of physical play. If you never had a chance to play sports and games as a child, however, now is the time to begin. In the immortal words of a California T-shirt: IT'S NEVER TOO LATE TO HAVE A HAPPY CHILD-HOOD

No Time, No Money

Spare time is about as scarce as spare change these days. And both tend to be particularly unavailable to women. Women still earn considerably less than men, with forty-seven percent of single female parents living below the poverty line. And despite any media blather about men who do their share of household chores, most women who have male partners still spend considerably more time cooking, doing laundry, and cleaning the toilet bowl than their partners do, even when they have full-time jobs. When your time is taken up by work and child care, and your money goes for the necessities, exercise can get bumped to a low rung on the priority ladder. If we categorized exercise as "medical expenses" (or the prevention thereof) instead of "leisure-time activity," it might make it to a higher rung, but that still would not change the reality that exercising costs time and money, and that both are in short supply for women.

For the least expensive form of exercise beneficial to health, brisk walking or running, a pair of shoes that will provide adequate support costs between $30 and $100. If you want to go to dance or other classes, costs average between $2 and $10 per class, depending on where you live. If you want to join a gym or club, costs generally range from a few hundred to as high as a few thousand dollars. Buying any additional exercise clothing or equipment adds to the total, as does child care if that is necessary.

When you consider that the minimum time necessary for exercise to achieve an optimal fitness effect is between one and a half to three hours per week (at thirty minutes per day, three to six days per week) it doesn't sound like a lot. But when you add the time for traveling to and from an exercise location, showering, and changing clothes, the total may be very considerable indeed. Given that many women still harbor the feeling it is "wrong" to take time for themselves, particularly if it is for enjoyment and does not include their families, then it's a wonder there are any women out there exercising at all. But there are, because, as you know, women are truly amazing.

When you consider the demands that compete for your time and money, you must make exercise a top priority, a self-care necessity, for you to have any hope of doing it on a regular basis. Too many other priorities may intervene if you leave doing it to chance. Most women find it helpful to put exercise into their schedules at a specific time on a specific day. Interestingly enough, if you do manage to achieve a regular exercise schedule, you are likely to become hooked on it, at which point you will stick to it come hell or high water. Many women have developed such a commitment to being active that if they can't find or afford child care, they take their kids with them on walks or share child care with other active moms. A few exercise classes provide child care, and some progressive companies provide time and facilities for exercise in the work place. While still woefully inadequate to meet the needs of active women, efforts in this direction could make an active life-style more accessible to all women. We can join together to encourage such progress. But for now, take whatever time you can for exercise and don't feel guilty either about taking the time or not taking as much time as you think you should.

For some women the lack of money can be an even more serious barrier to exercise, and all the motivation in the world will not change that. But it is also well to keep in mind that while women have statistically less income than men, we are the prime supporters of a weight-loss industry that racks up billions in profits every year. Most of us have probably wasted money on some "miracle cure." We could have bought more long-term rewards with the money we have spent on weekly weight-loss classes, diet books, pills, and other products, not to mention all the cosmetic products that go to work on the surface and leave the true sources of health, hence beauty, untouched.

While larger women certainly should have as much freedom as smaller women to plunge into beauty-products-land, if you have concluded that exercise is too expensive, you should take a close look at how you spend both your money and your time to see whether the long-term benefits are going to you rather than to the weight-loss and cosmetics industries. There is no substitute for the healthy glow that comes from good circulation, the graceful sureness that comes from exercised muscles and reflexes, and the relaxed self-confidence that a comfortable body exudes. All of these benefits come not from beauty treatments but from regular exercise, particularly exercise that stretches your imagination about your abilities and builds confidence in your body from the inside out. Exercise is a way to make a long-term investment in yourself. To repeat a well-worn advertising phrase, "And I'm worth it!"

Do You Have It in My Size?

For years the answer to this question was a maddening and humiliating *no*. For some unfathomable reason it was as if large women were invisible to the designers. We were forced to buy any old thing we could squeeze into, regardless of whether we liked it. And that was true for "regular" clothes—exercise clothing was simply nonexistent.

At long last clothing manufacturers are getting hip to the fact that human beings come in all sizes and that millions of those sizes are big ones. It is large women themselves who deserve a lot of the credit for starting businesses to meet the clothing needs of larger women. No longer do we have to suffer through polyester pant suits and ill-fitting, dull-colored, unfashionable, overpriced sack dresses. Clothing that fits, is comfortable, and meets the needs of whatever activity you are doing is a basic necessity for the active woman. There is nothing more distracting than worrying about whether you are going to split your seams if you do a particular movement. But it's not just a question of being able to buy clothes that make movement possible. Like everyone else, we want clothes that help make us feel good about ourselves. A new, just-right piece of comfortable exercise-wear can be just the incentive you need to get out there and enjoy yourself.

While it is true that clothing is much more accessible now than

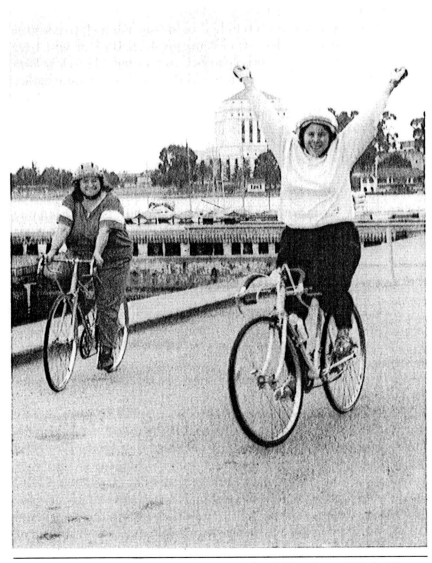

Michelle Dethke can exclaim, "Look, Ma, no hands!" as she and Linda Minor bicycle around Oakland's Lake Merritt.

it used to be, we still have a long way to go. Rural women have to travel to bigger cities or rely on catalogues, and very large women still have considerable trouble finding their size. While dance leotards are now more accessible in wild and beautiful prints and colors, most exercise clothing is still scarce or totally unavailable in sizes over 18 or 20. Will someone please take heed and make stretch cycling pants, one hundred percent cotton sweats, bathing suits for active swimmers, and waterproof hiking gear in big sizes? As greater numbers of large women become more active, these items may become more accessible for all of us. Keep in mind that there is nothing like consumer demand to increase supply—all manufacturers like to make money—so make your clothing needs known. Someday this barrier to activity may vanish completely! In the meantime, check out the clothing manufacturers in the appendix.

Bounding Over Barriers

According to Hopi Indian tradition, "Running lifts the heart, dispels sadness, firms up the flesh, and renews one's vigor." We could all benefit from the wisdom of this Hopi tradition since surely we could all use a lift in our spirits and renewed energy to live our lives as we choose. We non-Indians could also benefit from the wisdom of Indian people when considering the issue of respect.

In some American Indian tribes many people are prone to great weight; thus they, like the rest of us, must endure the medical establishment's efforts to force conformity to "ideal" weight charts. Dieting is no stranger in Indian communities, and it has not worked for them either. But Indian people do not make matters even worse for themselves by attaching a social stigma to body size. As in many cultures of the world, large-sized bodies are common, and respect has nothing to do with size but is based instead on character and actions. Some of the most fearless and outspoken tribal leaders are women, many of them large women, and they certainly don't wait for respect to be "given" to them. They assume respect as a given in their lives and get on with the business of improving the health of their communities. If all large women lived with such a strong sense of self-respect and determination, we would all be far healthier as a result.

The remainder of this book is dedicated to helping you learn to enjoy your body for what it can do, not continue to castigate it or to see it as the barrier to a healthier, more active life. Now that you've had a chance to get a bit more comfortable with the idea of fat *and* fit, and have begun to plan how to bound over some of the barriers that actually can stand in your way (you *have* begun bounding, right?), we'll go on to the nuts and bolts of getting out there and working up a sweat.

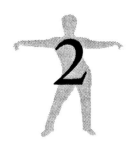

Getting Started

A Different Approach

So you're intrigued, you're enthusiastic, maybe even fired up. You're ready to run out, join a $500 health club, and make a chart for the refrigerator. You're gonna whip that body into shape! Well, stop right there. Does all this sound familiar? You've been here before.

Consider the last time you tread this ground. It's time to sort out what you can use in this approach from what trips you up.

Most of us try to make changes in our lives by force of willpower. We see our present state as unacceptable and resolve to control it. Today we are bad; tomorrow we will be perfect. Today we are a pallid "before"; tomorrow, after we spend $500 to join a health club and another $100 on aerobic gear, we will be a glowing "after." Does any of this sound familiar?

Do you know anyone who has made a change lasting more than six months this way? Most often, willpower eventually gives way to rebellion. For every action there is an equal and opposite reaction. This is because we usually have mixed feelings. Every change in our lives, even seeming improvements, implies the end of what is—the death of the familiar. And when the natural resistance to change is coupled with contempt for who we are until we change, some insulted part of us asserts itself by sabotaging that change.

If this seems accurate to you, if you have witnessed in yourself and in others the inevitable failure of the willpower strategy over the long haul, would you be willing to try a different tack? The first step in making modest, long-term change instead of dramatic, short-term change is to stop trying to reject the self you have in favor of an ideal, perfect self. To do this it is helpful to realize that you're already doing some of what you want to do and that you're a fine person right now and will continue to be a fine person even if you throw this book out the window.

We seem to be more willing to perform for the carrot than the stick. Something intrigues you about this idea of movement. What made you pick up this book? What curiosity, fantasy, yearning has kept you reading this far? What do you want?

Understanding Your Agenda

It does not have to be a big leap from where you are to where you want to be. You are probably more active than you realize. Do you carry your grocery bags into your home? Climb stairs at work? Keep up with children? Spend a few hours walking through the local department store or shopping mall? Your body doesn't know the difference between lifting grocery bags, children, and barbells. And because you weigh more, every movement you make can be considered a greater workout. Don't laugh: As a way of increasing their strength, athletes have been known to work out in rubber body suits with pockets that fill with water.

You already respond to your body's "hunger to move" without thinking about it. You tap your foot impatiently in the checkout line after having to stand still for fifteen minutes. You begin to bounce your knees after half an hour of watching TV. You even shift around in bed while you sleep. Next time you find yourself fidgeting, notice that your body is asking for release into movement—and start thinking about what kind of movement it would most enjoy.

Getting in Touch with the Itch to Move

This is a relaxation and visualization exercise designed to help you get to know your desire to move. It is easier to do if you either have someone you trust read slowly to you while you close your eyes or tape-record yourself reading slowly and replay it with your eyes closed.

You can do this exercise more than once; in fact, it can be a daily practice to help you identify what sort of movement you want.

First, lie down on a comfortable surface and loosen any constricting clothing so you can relax and breathe. Gently close your eyes and let your attention come to rest on your breathing. You are not trying to change your breathing, you are just noticing it, trusting that after all this time your breathing can take care of itself. In and out, in and out, let the rhythm lull you.

Imagine the path of your breath as it comes into your body, warming your insides. It flows through your nose, down your throat, into your lungs. You can imagine that it keeps flowing down, warming your stomach, your pelvis, and radiating into your arms and legs, all the way to the tips of your fingers and toes.

Your breath washes through the blocked places in your body, and as you breathe out, it takes with it any tension. Like an ocean wave, it brings in warmth and nourishment, and takes out waste and tension. Feel the waves flowing in and out for a few minutes.

Now begin at your feet and check each part of your body. What would your feet like? Do your toes need to curl and stretch? Experiment with curling your toes tightly and then stretching them out and away from one another, then let them relax.

Move up to your ankles. Flex, then point your feet and circle them one way and then the other. What do your calves need? Do they feel itchy, wanting to be warmed in movement? Tense and hold them, then release. Move up to your knees and thighs. Often the big muscles in your thighs hunger to be moved. Make them hard and tight for a moment. Squeeze them and feel the pleasure of that warmth, then release.

Move to your buttocks. Tense one cheek, then the other, then both. Squeeze hard and hold, then release. Draw your attention to your abdominal muscles. Press your lower back down onto the surface you're lying on so there's no gap. Push down, down, then release. Feel the flow of relaxation moving up your body. Continue upward, squeezing your shoulder blades together tightly, and feel the pleasure of stretching, then release. Notice the feeling in your hands. Squeeze your fingers into tight fists, hold them for a moment, then relax and let your hands uncurl gently.

Finally, screw your face up tightly, pursing your lips, squeezing your eyes, and wrinkling your nose and forehead. Hold tightly, then release.

Your body is now warm and relaxed. What sort of movement do you see in your mind at this time? Try on a few ideas. Imagine how your muscles would feel doing something. Slow and easy? Or do you need something stronger, something to pump heat? Smooth, fluid motion? Or harder, tighter movements? Where in your body do you feel a readiness for hard work? Take a few moments to localize your desire.

Do you want this activity to be in water or on land? Do you want to move to music? Do you want fast or slow pacing? Steady or a variety? Do you want to be alone or with friends? Let your imagination call on every sense to paint a picture for you.

What do you see? What do you hear? What fragrance is in the air? Who is there?

Give yourself a few minutes to really embellish the scene.

When you feel ready, let your attention return to your breath. Then slowly open your eyes.

You might want to write down your impressions and thoughts, or you can just reflect on what you envisioned.

The purpose is to take the time to check in with your physical self and get to know your feelings about movement. The exercise is only one method of doing this and will be more helpful to some people than others. If you try the same exercise again, you may have a different experience. But if nothing much happens for you after several attempts, you might simply ask yourself direct questions about what sort of movement appeals to you.

During the visualization you may or may not have felt any relaxation. You may or may not have wanted movement. You may or may not have seen yourself engaged in any physical activity. In this sort of exercise there are no right or wrong responses. In fact, for some people the most powerful message they get from doing this exercise is a fear of any kind of physical movement. Many of us have had painful feelings about our bodies, and sometimes this is the reason we would prefer to "live above the chin" and ignore the rest. Doing an exercise that puts you in touch with your body can also put you in touch with these long-buried emotions. If this happens for you, treat yourself with compassion rather than contempt. You might like some comforting right now—a hug or a soothing bath or a talk with a trusted friend.

If you have discovered painful feelings, it is important to know that movement may be one of the things which can help heal that pain. Exercise can enable you begin to balance the litany of disappointments and embarrassments with feelings of pleasure and competence, coordination, and agility. But this is a slow and rocky journey. Give yourself time.

If you did come up with some images of the kind of movement

you wanted, it might have surprised you, given what you thought about yourself up to now. How can you use this information?

Location of the hunger.   If you felt your "itch to move" in your thigh muscles, you need something that will work those muscles. Brisk walking, cycling, jogging, nonimpact aerobics, or working out on a leg press will work your thighs. Lifting weights, racquet sports, calisthenics, and swimming can work your arms.

Type of movement.   Slow, easy movements are the norm in t'ai chi, yoga, and some kinds of ethnic dance. Harder, tighter movements are required for the martial arts or aerobics. What appealed to you at this time?

Environment.   Land or water sports? Alone or with companions? Individual or team? Do you want to hear an underwater stillness? The noisy commotion of a squash court? The pulsating rhythms of an aerobic dance class? Do you want the privacy of your own thoughts? The companionship of a close friend? The heat of a full-out competition? Use this information to help you choose among the endless variety of ways to move.

Getting in Touch with Your Fears

You may now have a better idea about what sort of movement you'd like, but it's equally important to get an idea about your resistances to movement—the fears, concerns, distaste, and turnoffs you experience when you think about it. And don't assume that such resistances prove you're a born couch potato. Everyone has them, just as everyone has the counter-urge to move. The important thing is to find out what your negative feelings are and then figure out which of them are realistic and what you can do to make things easier on yourself. Some of the worries you have may seem silly or ridiculous, but for the moment you have to suspend judgment in order to see what they are.

You might take a sheet of paper and divide it into two columns. Under the "Concerns" column, list whatever fears and anxieties pop into your head. Don't censor yourself. List everything. After a few minutes, when your pencil slows down, start a second column entitled "What I Can Do About Them." Consider whether there is something concrete you can do to render each of these concerns unnecessary. If so, write it down. For example, one of your concerns might be that you'll break a leg. A possible solution is to engage only in low-impact activities such as swimming where that risk is minimized. Or you may worry that people will laugh at you if they see you jogging. That concern may be minimized by jogging in a more private location or with friends.

There are significant barriers for the large woman who wants to become more active. We discussed some of them in Chapter 1, and we'll get to others in Chapter 9. In any case, understand that there may be some things you will not be able to do much about. If there are no activities designed for large women in your area, you lack that resource until you organize one. If there are bigoted people you can't avoid, you'll probably be exposed to nasty remarks. Your attitude toward yourself in these circumstances needs to be charitable so that at least you will not add insult to injury by berating yourself for things outside your control. As you become more confident in your right to be who you are, to live with respect for the body you have and to join with other like-minded women, the attitudes of others will be less likely to stop you from doing what you want and having a good time doing it.

Setting Goals

If the idea of setting goals reminds you of tired rituals like charts for the refrigerator door and two-sizes-too-small dresses waiting in the closet, you're not alone. Most of us have set weight-loss goals for ourselves in the form of charts, promises, deals, bets, rewards and/or punishments. Some of us are just too jaded by failures in the past to engage in any kind of behavioral goal-setting anymore and need to focus on the here-and-now unfolding of our desire for exercise. But if this is not the case for you, and you think it would help you to structure time in your schedule for movement, we have some suggestions about how to set goals that are reachable this time.

What makes a goal reachable? Let's say you have a generalized overall goal of improved health and fitness. How will you know when you get there? Well, you could take starting and interim measurements of your blood pressure or your resting pulse rate, which are measures of fitness. But you can make the goal even more reachable by anchoring it in behavior rather than results; for example, you might decide that during the next six months you will try at least one new movement activity that you have never tried before. You're going to do something you know is possible and define it in such a way that you can be clear about whether or not you have in fact done it. If you succeed then you have evidence that you can carry out your intentions.

The most important aspect of setting goals is to do what you want to do. We are all well schooled in the art of people-pleasing, changing our wants to fit someone else's idea of how we should "improve" ourselves. We can comply for only so long; then, in some ornery, resentful, or overburdened moment, we throw the whole plan out the window. Instead, you can begin exploring what gives you satisfaction. Your goals will be as individual as you are. Allow yourself time to be still and listen to your heart about what you want, and then set goals that help you achieve it.

Whether you set goals or not, you will undoubtedly observe your progress along the way. There are hundreds of baby steps involved in any lasting change, which is an easy fact to lose sight of in our "before and after" culture. That either/or thinking is everywhere: Who has not, as a grown woman, described herself as "good" or "bad" depending on her diet and exercise behavior that day? The truth is there is no "before" or "after," only "during." As long as we are alive we are in process.

Rather than viewing physical activity as an either/or choice, draw yourself a continuum. The diagram below moves from "contemplating your navel" at one extreme to "running marathons" at the other. Between them are many steps along the way to increased physical activity and awareness. These are just suggestions that may inspire you. You will notice that each of the steps involves specific behavior rather than vaguely defined improvement.

0	1	2	3	4	5	6	7	8	9	10	11	12	13	14	15

Mary   Martha
Meditator   Marathoner

1. Throwing away the TV remote control and getting up to change the channel.

2. Walking around the house at each half-hour break between TV programs. Learning to take your resting pulse.

3. Walking across the street to visit a neighbor instead of calling on the telephone. Sharing your goal of trying to be more active and enlisting her support.

4. Parking your car at the far end of the grocery store parking lot. Buying a book about an inspiring woman or an activity you want to learn more about.

5. Getting off the bus three blocks away from your stop and walking the extra distance.

6. Going for a half-hour walk before or after supper twice a week. Taking up Ping-Pong for fun.

7. Doing stretching and strengthening exercises for your back fifteen minutes a day, three times a week. Developing an awareness of where in your body you hold tension.

8. Doing We Dance exercises and dance steps once a week at home. Learning to calculate your aerobic pulse rate.

9. Expanding your walks to include a hike with a friend. Taking lots of deep breaths of fresh air. Having a dance party.

10. Finding a martial arts, belly dancing, or yoga class. Buying a bicycle and riding it. Starting a swim group with a few friends.

11. Buying good jogging shoes and a book to explain the basics, and beginning to alternate walking and jogging on your outings.

12. Expanding your treks to include entering a local walk-a-thon for a good cause. Luxuriating in a hot bath, sauna, or Jacuzzi afterwards.

13. Enrolling your daughter in the sport/dance/exercise class of her choice. Taking her on weekend hikes. Getting a massage for yourself.

14. Beginning to train for a five- or ten-kilometer race several months in advance. Visualizing yourself crossing the finish line while running. Expanding your back exercises to include leg work and all-around stretching.

15. Finishing a race. Performing a dance. Looking for ways to have even more fun, smile more, and learn more about your body. Giving yourself credit for all your victories. Refusing to engage in any self-abusing internal dialogue. Looking in the mirror and saying, "I am healthy and strong," and meaning it!

Even when using a continuum it is easy to see one end as bad and the other as good and, by association, to see yourself as bad if you contemplate your navel and good if you run marathons. Whether you exercise or not is unrelated to your worth as a person, but if you decide you want more movement in your life, you should realize that you'll probably be able to do some things some of the time but not everything every day. Change occurs in stages and is just as significant at the beginning as at the end. After all, to finish a race you have to start it. And then you have to decide what to do next!

Many Paths to the Same Goal

The exploratory exercises presented so far are probably new to just about everyone and are only one way to get going. What did folks do before we wrote this book? We asked some of the women in the We Dance class, all of them over two hundred pounds, about how they started exercising and how they keep movement in their busy lives.

Robin: How did I start exercising? I swam competitively as a teenager. There was a swim for large women, and I started going to that. Although I didn't do laps, just being in the water on a regular basis made my body want to move more. So my friend Cheryl and I searched for an exercise class for large women, and we finally found this. It was really hard for me in the beginning because I was not physically competent. I could do only half the class for a long time, and it was a year before I did every single repetition. I just had to *want* it a lot. My body wanted to move, but I had to prevent my ego from getting in the way and let it be okay that I wasn't very good at what I was doing. These days, if someone asks me, "Do you want to go out to dinner on Monday night?" I say, "No, I have a dance class on Monday nights."

Gloria: I've always been large. I always could dance, and I've always enjoyed it. I was never hiding inside myself, but after I had my two children, I gained a lot of weight. I wasn't able to take it off, and my self-confidence plummeted. I tried going to one of those weight-training places, where all those skinny little women bounced around, but I didn't feel very comfortable. My mother told me about We Dance, and the rest is history. I have one thing to say about showing up all the time. I have trouble doing that because of the other commitments in my life, but what I find important is not to quit trying. I drop out and don't come for a while and have problems making it for a lot of different reasons, but the important thing is telling myself, "Well, forget it and start over. Just keep doing it." It's not even a goal of doing it until I get it right. It's just coming when I can. It's helped me enormously. I feel a lot better, and my confidence is better. Even my husband's attitude has changed a lot!

Frances: When you want to get started in any kind of a group, yes, it's important that you have a commitment to do this every week, but it's even more important that you do this with a buddy so you have someone to go with. Otherwise it's too easy not to feel up to it some Monday night, if you're the only one who's affected. But if you have to give a ride to somebody else or even if it's just that she's expecting you, it makes it a whole lot harder not to go.

Ruth: I started the class because I wanted the physical benefits. I was living at home, looking for a job, and I wasn't doing anything active. My 120-pound mother does an aerobics class four days a week, and I thought, heck, I can do that too! I was only twenty-five or twenty-six, and I thought, "It's really stupid for me to be out of shape at my age because if I don't get in shape now, it's going to be harder when I get older."

So I went. And I scared myself. I pushed myself pretty hard, and I was exhausted and sore. I thought, "God, you're really out of

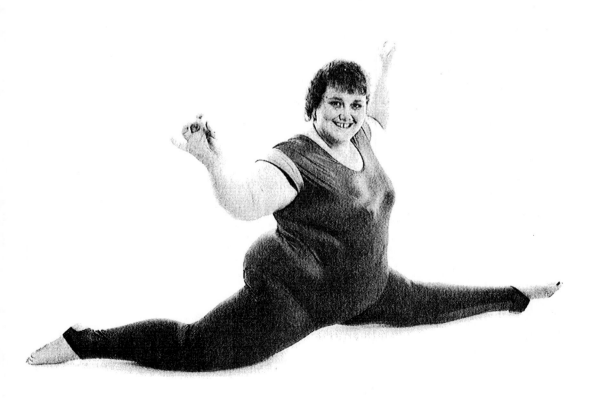

Carol Squires dazzles her *We Dance* friends.

shape! This is really bad!" And so I went the next time and took it a little bit easier. I wore shoes, which helped, and I wasn't sore and felt really positive. I thought, "Well, gee, it's two classes, and already you're feeling better about the way you move." And after about three or four weeks, I said, "Wow! I feel better all the time. I feel better when I'm walking down the street. My posture's better, and I'm not sore at the end of the day. I feel healthier and more vital."

I notice when I don't go to class for about three weeks my back feels stiff, and that's one of the things that gets me to go to class even when I'm feeling down or don't want to be around other people. I think, "Well, if you don't go, you're going to feel terrible." And that helps.

Once I felt more comfortable, I started looking at the people I was dancing with. I saw a lot of women who were a lot larger than I was who were still attractive, successful, vital people. I thought, "You can be a large woman and be attractive and have a successful job. It's not as if your size has to be a limit on what you can accomplish."

Listening to these women, it becomes clear that when it comes right down to it, getting started requires a leap of faith. No one came to We Dance without doubts. Some people brought friends as supports, and some found friends in the class. And if they were able to suspend judgment about the things that were difficult and able to delight in the parts that were easy, their confidence grew and spread to other areas of their lives.

We hope you've found the recommendations in this chapter— the relaxation exercise, the concerns list, the goal-setting continuum, and the inspirational words of others like yourself—useful. The important thing is that you have taken the time to think about what you want to do. You have been willing to try approaching this subject from a new angle, from inside rather than outside. Congratulations! You've taken the most important step—the first one.

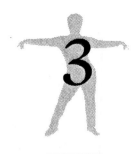

3

Exercise and Weight

Separating Fact from Propaganda

In the last chapter we talked about how to discover your own feelings about exercise. Such techniques can be used by anyone who wishes to become more active. Now we will focus on information about exercise for large bodies in particular.

First are questions concerning exercise's effect on weight: Does exercise result in weight loss? What happens physically when you exercise? How does a large body differ from an average-sized body in the way it uses fuel?

Next we focus on weight's effect on exercise, that is, the special challenges of being a large person beginning to exercise: What effect does moving more weight have on your exertion level? Your physical safety?

We complete the discussion by exploring the practical aspects of being a large person beginning to exercise: How do you get the most out of a health examination? Where can you find appropriate clothing? How do you adapt a regular class to your needs or start one just for large women? No matter what kind of activity you decide to do, this chapter gives you a foundation of information about your body and how it will respond to exercise.

There are still many unresearched questions in the general area of exercise and weight, and at the outset it is important to stress that this field is full of controversy and contradiction. We do not have the final answers to any of these questions. What we will try to do is outline the broad picture.

The first question to address is the effect of exercise on weight. Most of us are familiar with the idea that our bodies use calories—stored energy—to meet the physical demands of life. We have been told to count the calories going in and estimate the calories going out (for basic metabolism plus the specific activities of the day). On the basis of these calculations we can figure out how much weight we should expect to gain or lose.

One problem with that model is that it does not consider the efficiency with which we use up the calories coming in. Apparently there is a wide variety of rates at which people burn calories, so much so that a 120-pound and a 220-pound woman can each maintain their weights on exactly the same diet! It is as if the 220-pound woman is a fuel-efficient car, getting many more miles to the gallon than her "gas-guzzling" thinner friend.

Second, there seems to be a regulatory function that each of our bodies performs to maintain our weight within a narrow range, regardless of variations in the number of calories we consume on different days. Observations to this effect have led researchers to propose a new model of how humans maintain, gain, and lose weight, called the setpoint theory. This is a more complex model than the more linear calories in/calories out model.

Setpoint Theory

Consider the following experiments:

In 1944* a group of men was put on starvation rations for six months. They lost one fourth of their body weight, became lethargic and miserable, and developed food obsessions. The experimenters increased their rations slightly, and the subjects immediately began to gain weight. At the end of the restricted period, when they were allowed to eat freely, they ate ravenously until they regained their original weights, at which point they began eating normal amounts again. (Sound familiar to any dieters out there?)

In the mid sixties another researcher did a study in which a

---

*For all references, see William Bennett's and Joel Gurin's book, *Dieter's Dilemma* (New York: Basic Books, 1982).

group of men were overfed until they gained twenty percent of their starting weights. The participants needed to eat much more than predicted—an average of two thousand extra calories a day—to put on and maintain that additional weight. The men were lethargic and passive at their peak weights. Once the experiment was over, they spontaneously ate half their normal diets until they returned to their original weights.

A starving body gains weight when given a little bit more food, while an overfed body drops weight when given a little bit less food—and in neither case do "calories in" appear to equal "calories out." Moreover, what is "starving" and what is "overfed" is not what we commonly think of as thin or fat. It is rather the relationship of one's current weight to the weight you were born to maintain. Setpoint theory can account for all of the above. It is based on the idea that each person's body has an individual "setting" for weight and tends to maintain that weight, the same way that a thermostat maintains the set temperature in a house. Our metabolism will compensate for what we eat by burning hotter or cooler (using up calories faster or slower) to maintain that setting. Setpoint theory is the most elegant way of explaining why our bodies seem to be "invested" in maintaining a certain amount of fat; why most fat people can eat the same amount (or less) than thin people and stay fat; why some thin people can eat a great deal and fail to gain any weight; and why almost everyone maintains a fairly consistent weight (whether over, at, or below the "ideal" weight charts) without consciously counting calories.

We have been wrong to assume that all bodies have been "set" to conform to the "ideal" height/weight charts. In fact, the bodies of dieting fat people behave as if they are starving—that is, they conserve energy even if the charts say they are "overweight." Researchers are beginning to notice that people who have been fat most of their lives and who temporarily diet down to their "ideal" weight sometimes exhibit symptoms similar to those of anorexics: obsessive thoughts about food, difficulty staying warm, low blood pressure, and so on. We can see easily that the anorexic's body is starving; what we haven't known until now is that bodies which appear to be normal or even above average in weight can also be starving. Starving takes on a new meaning. Rather than being below the "ideal" weight, it means being below one's own biological weight setting. Apparently setpoints can differ widely from person to person. Some set for fat, some set for thin, most set for in-between, but for any one individual, the setpoint is essentially fixed.

Setpoint theory's explanation as to why diets fail puts the blame on metabolism, not willpower. It seems that the dieter's body responds to reduced calories as though it were being starved. Hence the metabolism slows down to conserve energy. The body becomes more efficient and stops losing fat. To keep losing fat, one would have to continually decrease caloric intake, and each decrease would result in a further slowing of the metabolism. The physical and health effects of such metabolic shifts are not well understood at this point.

What determines the setpoint setting? No one knows, but it is probable that heredity plays an important role. New research shows that identical twins reared apart will attain nearly identical weights; in fact, weight is more likely than height to turn out the same! Environmental factors may modify an individual's setpoint: sweet (even artifically sweet) and fatty foods, as well as a diet with a great variety of foods, seem to raise it; nicotine, amphetamines, and physical activity seem to lower it moderately. Of course, lowering your setpoint by taking speed, smoking cigarettes, and eating only one kind of food all day will lead you to an early grave. Laboratory rats exposed to smoke and fed only rat chow may be thinner, but if they could speak, they'd surely tell you it's a short and brutish life. There may be other factors that affect setpoint which haven't been discovered yet, but in the meantime, good nutrition (*not* dieting) and rousing physical activity seem to offer some promise.*

All dieters have experienced the depressing experience of "plateauing" at a given weight, feeling lethargic and cranky, straying from the diet, and immediately putting the weight back on—often even adding a few pounds. Setpoint theory explains this phenomenon as your body shifting into "starvation mode." It becomes extremely efficient with each morsel and slows down, metabolically speaking, to conserve energy. Few people with much self-esteem can choose this kind of life for long, and most will return to eating normally. The slowed-down metabolism continues to be overly efficient at conserving calories and therefore returns you to your original weight very quickly, sometimes even overshooting by a few pounds for insurance. Most people feel psychologically depressed for having failed, and physically a little heavier, and the cycle begins again with the next dieting attempt.

With any given attempt at dieting, your weight returns pretty

---

*For more information check *Jane Brody's Nutrition Book A Lifetime Guide to Good Eating for Better Health and Weight Control* (New York: Bantam Books, 1982). Jane Brody advises eating a variety of whole foods and lowering your overall intake of dietary fat, salt, caffeine, and alcohol.

much to normal, but after repeated attempts your body may become more lethargic and even heavier. Moreover, with diets under about twelve hundred calories a day, your body uses up not only fat but also muscle tissue, water, and even bone mass for fuel. When you put the weight back on, however, it is in the form of water and fat. Thus, the scale may show your original weight, but a higher percentage of it is now fat.

How do you tell what your setpoint is? The easy answer is that it is the weight you always come back to after you stop trying to "control" your eating. But chronic dieters may have trouble remembering a time when they didn't try to control their eating. Those of us who have spent years going back and forth between eating weighed portions of "legal" foods and ravenously bingeing find it difficult to know what it feels like to eat in response to physical hunger. If you can stop dieting long enough to end the starvation-binge cycle, you may find yourself losing some weight. That's because the diet-binge method of eating often results in your eating more than your body is physically hungry for. Eating more than your body is hungry for can raise your weight above the setpoint. You can only tell where your setpoint is if you eat when you are physically hungry and stop when you are physically satisfied. People who aren't compulsively dieting/eating but are fairly inactive may also moderately lower their setpoints by increasing physical activity. But it is quite possible to eat healthfully, get plenty of exercise, and still maintain a body weight that is over the "ideal" charts. It seems to be a genetic fact.

Setpoint theory liberates many of us from the damning and self-defeating notion that we are fat because we overeat and that all we need is a little more willpower to lose weight. For some of us this will be the idea that sets us free to live our lives without guilt or self-blame and without illusions of some size 10 future. But others of us will feel trapped and despairing at the notion that there is no hope of permanently losing weight. If going on diets just lowers the metabolism (and maybe ultimately makes us fatter) and exercise won't radically alter the setpoint, then what hope is there?

William Bennett, one of the authors of *Dieter's Dilemma,* was asked this question in a lecture, and he asked the audience whether they were depressed that they couldn't spread their arms and fly: This, too, is a physical limitation. While it's true that this is little comfort to those who must live with daily social oppression, by saying that fatness is a biological fact Bennett brings us closer to a future in which society stops treating us as if our body size is the result of psychological weakness. In many other cultures fat people lead healthy, happy, and satisfying lives; nothing inherent in fat precludes these things.

Aerobic Exercise

How does exercise affect the setpoint?

Exercise seems to moderately lower the setting, but only for as long as you maintain that level of activity in your life. One of the great advantages of exercise, as opposed to dieting, is that it does not cause the starvation response described above; in other words, your metabolism does not slow down to conserve body weight. If you think of dieting and exercise as two forms of treatment, dieting has many undesirable side effects—slowed metabolic rate, sluggishness, loss of muscle mass, feelings of deprivation—which exercise does not share. In fact, exercise seems to have the opposite effects: heightened metabolic rate, both during and for some time after exercise; increased energy and muscle mass; and feelings of well-being. While most people hate dieting, lots of people learn to love movement.

There are two kinds of exercise, aerobic and anaerobic. These terms describe the two different ways your body meets its need for fuel when you're exerting yourself. A short, intense burst of exertion, such as weight lifting and sprinting, is called "anaerobic." The body uses the sugar (glycogen) present in muscle tissue for this type of demand. In contrast, sustained, moderately intense exertion, such as bicycling, swimming, and aerobic dance, is called "aerobic" (literally, "with air"). Your body uses fat deposits to meet this type of demand. It needs the presence of oxygen to convert fat to energy, and it gets this from the deep breathing you do during aerobic exercise.

It is aerobic exercise that affects the setpoint setting. This is very important to know if you have dieted a lot in the past. Research is beginning to suggest that people with a long history of dieting (whether successful at producing weight loss or not) have slowed down their metabolic rate considerably. It is as if the body learns with each starvation to be more efficient with food. People who are already genetically "gifted" at making the most of their food—that is, people who stay fat on an average amount of food—will become even more efficient as a result of dieting. In contrast, aerobic exercise seems to prime the body to waste calories. It heats up the metabolic rate so that you continue to burn calories even after you've stopped exercising.

While there are clear benefits, aerobic exercise is not a surefire way to lose weight. If it were, people would do it, get thin, and the billion-dollar dieting industry would dry up and blow away. No matter what you do, if you are a genetically large person, you will not turn into a genetically thin person. But if you find something you like to do enough that you keep doing it, your body will certainly become more firm, sleek, strong, and capable. Most people find that because exercise builds muscle and uses fat, and because muscle tissue weighs more than fat, their bodies streamline even though the scale reads the same or more.

Because muscle tissue weighs more than fat, the scale gives only a crude and often misleading indication of fatness. Fitness consultants recently have begun using techniques to measure body fat instead of just weight, such as underwater (hydrostatic) weighing, bioelectrical impedance, and calipers. All of these technologies are designed to measure the percentage of body weight that is fat versus what is lean body mass (bone, muscle, and fluid). As you might expect, there are now "ideal body fat percentages" to replace the "ideal weight" charts, and they are about as scientific! Essentially what the fitness industry has done is come up with the typical body fat percentages of average folks as well as the typical body fat percentages of athletes, and then suggest that the ideal is somewhere in between. This line of reasoning seems to go as follows: Athletes are healthy; athletes have low body fat percentages; therefore it is healthy to have low body fat percentages. What about all the other healthy people with higher body fat percentages? We really don't know enough to set an "ideal" body fat percentage.

If you want to assess the effect of exercise on your body, however, these fat-measuring techniques tell you more than the scale. If you are building muscle mass and replacing fat, the number on the scale may not go down but your body fat percentage probably will. You won't need technology to tell you that your clothes fit differently or that you can feel newly defined muscles or that—best of all—you are moving with new grace and competence. The joy and ease of movement will help you make peace with your body at any size.

Finding Your Target Heart Rate

While anaerobic exercise is useful for building strength, aerobic exercise builds stamina by conditioning your cardiovascular system, that is, making your heart and lungs more efficient. Using the large muscle groups in your legs and buttocks challenges your heart to pump more blood, faster. You feel the evidence of this in your increased heartbeat rate.*

Many different activities can be aerobic: a brisk walk, swimming laps, going out to dance, skating, and so on. In all of these cases the demand on your body is enough to make you breathe deeply for a sustained period of time without becoming breathless. Most of us understand that aerobic exercise requires us to boost our exertion level, but we rarely think that we can also boost it *too* high. Large people especially need to be aware that trying to keep up with activities paced for 120-pound bodies may push you above the target range. It is the "middle zone" of exertion that produces the greatest benefits.

To determine whether you have reached but not exceeded that middle zone, check your pulse. You can find your pulse either at your neck or at your wrist (see page 92). Usually the pulse is stronger at the neck. Place your index finger on your adam's apple and slide it toward the corner of your jaw. About halfway to the hinge in your jaw there is a little soft spot. This is where your carotid artery is. The second spot for checking your pulse is the radial artery in your wrist. Lay your wrist, palm up, in your other palm. Curl your fingers around your wrist like a bracelet. Let your fingertips rest in the soft groove between the middle and the thumb side of your wrist, and you should be able to feel your pulse.

Finding your pulse gets easier with practice. It is also easier to feel after you've been exerting yourself because your heartbeat is stronger. You might want to check your heart rate not only when you are exercising but also when you first wake up in the morning (resting pulse) and after your cool-down period after aerobic exercise (recovery pulse). As your heart and lungs become stronger and more efficient, your resting pulse becomes lower because your heart doesn't need to beat as often to do the same job. You will have to make your exercise more and more challenging to boost your heart rate into the aerobic range. After each exercise session, the more fit you become the quicker your heart rate will return to its resting pulse. So taking your pulse at all three times—resting, aerobically exercising, and recovering—will reveal your progress as you become more fit.

What number of beats per minute constitutes the aerobic

---

*There are other times that your heart rate may increase—for example, when you're frightened—that are not aerobic. There has to be an increased volume of blood pumping through your system, which happens by exerting the large muscle groups in your lower body.

range? You can find your target heart rate by using the following formula: Subtract your age from 220 and take sixty-five percent of the result (for the lower boundary of the target range) and eighty-five percent of the result (for the higher end). Here's the example for a thirty-year-old:

Step 1. 220 − 30 = 190
Step 2. 190 × .65 = 123.5 (lower end of target range)
Step 3. 190 × .85 = 161.5 (higher end of target range)

Thus a thirty-year-old's aerobic range is between 123 and 161 heartbeats per minute. As long as her rate remains in this range, she is exercising aerobically.

Practically speaking, you won't want to count your heart rate for a whole minute every time you stop to take your pulse. You will count for 6 seconds and then add a zero. For a thirty-year-old taking her pulse for 6 seconds, the aerobic range is between 12 and 16.

Let's try a second example, for a fifty-year old.

Step 1. 220 − 50 = 170
Step 2. 170 × .65 = 110.5 (lower end of aerobic range)
Step 3. 170 × .85 = 144.5 (higher end of aerobic range)

A fifty-year-old's aerobic range is between 110 and 144 beats per minute. If she is counting her pulse for 6 seconds, her target heart rate is between 11 and 14 beats.

When should you take your pulse? Anytime you want to get feedback on your body's response. In practice you will probably want to take your pulse midway through your exercise session to see if you are in the aerobic range; again at the end to confirm that you continued to exercise aerobically; and finally after a few minutes of cooling down to see that your heart rate has dropped toward its resting pulse. That first measurement is important because you can either step up the pace if your rate is below target or relax a little if it is above target, adjusting your pace in light of the information your body gives you.

After a period of time you will probably be able to tell subjectively whether you are exercising aerobically. You will be moving vigorously enough to breathe deeply and break into a sweat, but you should still be able to carry on a conversation. This is what Pat refers to in the coming chapters on sports as the "talk test."

Research shows that the minimum amount of exercise you can do and still maintain your current cardiovascular condition is 20 minutes at your aerobic pace, three times a week. To improve your condition, the minimum amount needed is about 25 to 30 minutes four times a week. But if you are just starting, any amount of activity will result in physical benefits, and it is important to make the change gradually. Taking your time gives your body and your schedule a chance to adapt.

Physical Safety

Now we come to the second series of questions that we raised in the beginning of this chapter: What is the effect of body weight on exercise? How is aerobic exercise different for larger bodies?

Picture yourself in the average aerobic class. The first consideration is that, in moving more weight, you are doing more physical work than your 110-pound neighbor. That means you are demanding more of your body, and your heart will work harder. The impor-

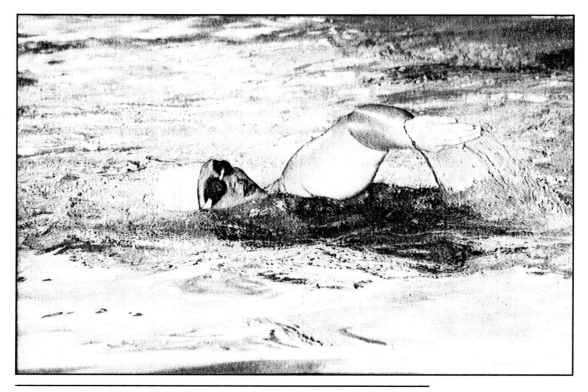

Swimming is the ideal aerobic activity for water lover Miriam Cantor.

tant question is whether your heart rate remains within your target range or whether, by trying to keep up with your neighbor, you have pushed it past that level. If it is too high, your heart and lungs will have trouble supplying your muscles with the fuel and oxygen they need. Contrary to the "harder is better" idea, this is the point of diminishing returns. It is important to note also that pushing your heartrate above the aerobic range may increase the risk of injury to your heart. The first number we calculated above—220 minus your age—is considered the maximum suggested heart rate, so you should consider that zone, between eighty-five and one hundred percent of your maximum heart rate, the "caution" zone. Your heart and lungs are laboring harder than necessary to build fitness, and you are heading for the outer limit of how fast your heart should beat under any circumstances. Classes paced for the 120-pound person to get her heart rate into the aerobic range are usually too fast for the 220-pound person.

The second consideration to take into account is the impact of your feet hitting the ground. Think about how many runners and other aerobic exercisers you know have ruined knees, shin splints, torn Achilles tendons, and damaged feet. Many people in the fitness industry have become concerned about the high rate of lower-body injuries for students and instructors, and are creating "low-impact" classes. In these activities one foot is always on the floor, which considerably lessens the bang. Another preventive step is to wear shoes with good padding across the ball of the foot. And the floor or playing surface is very important. It should have some "give" to it, like wood. Concrete floors, whether hidden by carpeting or not, are the worst.

If you find yourself in a high-impact aerobics class paced for 120-pound bodies, you may be able to protect yourself and get a good workout by transforming the high-impact steps into low-impact steps. This is doubly effective because it slows the pace as well as lessens the impact with which your feet meet the floor. To transform the steps, just remember to always keep one foot on the floor. A jogging step becomes a march, one-legged hops become knee lifts, and so on. Some high-impact steps are so complicated, their low-impact versions are hard to figure out. In that case you can simply march until the next one comes along. It's important to keep your legs moving so your heart rate stays up in the target range.

Finally, there are some movements that people with large breasts, stomachs, or thighs simply may not be able to do. You may be as flexible and strong as the next person, but you shouldn't have to choose between doing a proper sit-up and breathing! The pattern of strengths and weaknesses in your body might be different: Your legs might be stronger than your 110-pound neighbor's (after all, you are working out with weights every time you walk), but your abdominal muscles may be weaker. Or the fifth repetition of a leg lift tires you out more than your neighbor because she has less to lift. In all of these cases you need to trust your own body and see if the exercise can be tailored to your needs. If not, don't do it. You can always substitute an exercise you know to be safe and effective until the class moves on to an exercise you can do.

The problem with all of this advice about how to change the exercise class's movements to make them safe is that it requires you to do something that deviates from the rest of the class when you probably already feel deviant enough being the largest person there. Instructors can say, "Go at your own pace" until they are blue in the face, but students rarely feel comfortable about going slower when they need to. There is a subtle pressure in most classes to form a harmonious, lockstep tableau in the mirrors, like a precision marching band. But when your physical safety is at stake, sometimes you have to march to a different drummer or else find a different activity.

Because the average-sized person is considered the norm and most activities are geared for her, it is easy to feel that your body is distorted in some way. But really it is just different. Remember, for everyone but the thinnest and fattest person in the world, there is someone bigger and someone smaller than you. The range in the middle is vast compared with the range we see represented in a typical aerobics class. It's just arbitrary that in this country at this time exercise is geared to size 7's.

More Safety Basics

There are a few points that anyone who starts exercising should know. First, your body will be giving you all kinds of important feedback, in addition to your heart rate, about how exercise is affecting you. You might feel twinges, heat, fatigue, stretching sensations, and pain. It is important to understand what sort of feedback your body is giving you so you can act on it by continuing to exercise, slowing down the pace a bit, or stopping altogether, whichever is appropriate.

The heat you feel in your muscles after exerting them results from the buildup of lactic acid. It is not particularly harmful, but it causes discomfort, which is easily relieved by shaking the muscle out for a few seconds. Once you have shaken out, you can return to working the muscle with less discomfort.

Pain, on the other hand, means, "Pay attention, injury alert!" You might feel pain in a muscle, joint, or other location. In all cases, if you feel pain, you should stop what you're doing and hope you're not already injured. Ask your instructor, coach, or activities leader about what you're feeling; in the case of persistent pain, consult a sports medicine practitioner. The motto, "No pain, no gain," has caused needless suffering. Exercise does not have to hurt to be effective.

If you do pull or strain a muscle, the best first-aid treatments are rest, ice, compression, and elevation. Start them immediately. You should elevate the affected limb and wrap it, then apply crushed ice or a cold pack.* This will reduce swelling and inflammation, and give your body time to heal without further strain. Do not use heat for at least twenty-four hours, and even after that, don't apply localized heat such as a heating pad. Heat increases circulation to the injury site and causes swelling, which is what you are trying to avoid. Remember that this is just first-aid advice; the second part is following up with an examination of the injury by your medical practitioner. Don't hesitate to ask your practitioner whether this injury needs the attention of a specialist in sports medicine or a related discipline.

Other exercise basics include remembering to keep breathing properly and drinking plenty of fluids. There are exercises and movements in which your natural impulse is to hold your breath—sit-ups, for example. Just remember to breathe out on the exertion phase of the movement (for sit-ups, when you are raising yourself) and breathe in during the relaxation phase (when you are lowering yourself). Also, it is important to drink small amounts of water as you exercise. Your sense of thirst lags behind your actual need for water during exertion, so make a habit of drinking plenty of water, even when you're not feeling particularly thirsty. Because any type of aerobic exercise causes you to sweat, you may find that in addition to the water you drink during your workout you need to drink more

---

*Peak Condition, a sports medicine book by Dr. James Garrick (New York: Crown Publishers, 1986), gives detailed information about how to care for specific injuries and is worth having on hand.

water every day than you used to. The standard recommendation is to drink at least eight glasses of fluids per day.

So far you have looked inward to determine your own movement preferences. You've learned about the effects of exercise on weight and the effects of weight on exercise. You've picked up a few safety tips. Now it is time to get very practical and examine what else you need to know before launching yourself from the starting line.

If the preceding sections answered your questions about "what" and "why," this one tries to address nagging practical questions such as "Who?" "Where?" and "What can I wear?" Finding competent medical advice, clothes that fit, and a supportive, informed instructor at a good, safe facility can make your exercising life much easier.

Getting the Most from Your Health Checkup

Your reaction to the inevitable advice to see your doctor before starting an exercise program may well be: "No way!" Going to see a doctor is usually unpleasant for large people. There's the financial cost, often prohibitive for those who cannot get health insurance; the poorly concealed contempt and exasperation that many health care practitioners feel for the "obese"; and the monotonous, predictable advice to lose weight, regardless of the medical problem for which you sought treatment. And then there's the scale, the too-small paper robes that never close, and the overall feeling of being embarrassed and exposed in a hostile environment. It's no wonder you balk at the idea.

But somewhere out there is a competent and caring person who could work with you to minimize the risk of injury; to help you better understand your body's workings; to identify hidden weaknesses and strengths. To plunge ahead without this person as a partner is to give up your right to competent medical care and take an unknown and unnecessary risk. On the other hand, to try to find him or her is to make an investment in improving the quality of your health care and ultimately your life.

So how can you find this person without suffering through the rejects?

Decide what your requirements are. Does it matter whether the practitioner is male or female? Do you want a general practitioner for all your health needs, or do you want a specialist in sports medicine who has had specific training in risk assessment, exercise prescription, and injury rehabilitation? What about the cost of an evaluation?

Then see who's out there. Ask friends. Call your local National Association to Advance Fat Acceptance (NAAFA) chapter or women's center for a referral.* Check your community health clinic, which may have a sliding fee scale. Go to an event for large women (a fashion show, a performing group, a clothing store, and so forth) and ask whether anyone has found a good doctor. Look up the numbers of sports medicine specialists. Collect names and then call them.

Communicate your need for a thorough physical in preparation for increasing your physical activity level. What sort of services and expertise can s/he provide? How much will it cost? What is his/her attitude about large people?

You will probably come up with a range of services offered. This is because there is general disagreement about what procedures should be part of a pre-exercise medical examination. Some people believe a basic physical is enough while others contend you need a cardiac stress test, cholesterol level, and so forth. Still others maintain that the individual patient's health history should determine the diagnostic tests performed.

As usual, there are no easy answers. Are sports medicine physicians better helpers because they know more about exercise's effects on the human body? Or are they worse because they usually deal with lean, elite athletes? Are general practitioners better helpers because they see a range of problems and a range of patients? Or will they lack some specific knowledge? Controversy reigns in this area, but most experts maintain that in order to assess the risk of exercise one must undergo an examination revealing how your body responds to exertion, that is, a cardiac stress (or treadmill) test, and that the greater your practitioner's knowledge about sports medicine, the better.

Because health practitioners are human, inevitably there will be some way in which they are imperfect helpers. To make the most of this partnership it is important that you communicate your own needs and concerns clearly and promptly and that the practitioner be willing to learn what s/he doesn't already know or to refer you to someone who does.

---

*See the Appendix for more on NAAFA.

What to Wear

We asked the most avid shoppers we knew to research the activewear resources. Frances White and Robin Hopkins drew up a list of sources for sweats, T-shirts, leotards, tights, bras, shoes, and so forth (see Appendix). There are some disappointing gaps: still no one hundred percent cotton sweats or athletic uniforms, very little in super sizes, and limited availability or selection. But this year there was more than last year. We hope that's a trend!

Don't delay getting started because you want to buy special exercise gear. With the exception of having appropriate shoes, the fact that you are starting out at a low intensity means you probably don't need anything too specialized. This is your time to survey different activities to see what you like. It would be great if we could afford to be outfitted in top-of-the-line equipment for each different sport because there's no question that it adds to our skill, comfort, and safety. But unless money is no object, it is better to wait on the wardrobe until you know what activities you like best.

To get started you will probably be comfortable enough in anything you already own that allows for freedom of movement, is absorbent and breathable, and covers you for the times you're upside down and sideways! That could be a T-shirt, tank top, leotard, or sweat shirt, and sweatpants, parachute pants, or opaque tights (rather than nylons, which run and don't "breathe") and shorts.

Later, you may want to invest in aerobic wear. Originally leotards and tights were made of nylon, but the two newer fabrics that have replaced it are lycra and cotton-lycra blends. These represent a big step forward in comfort, support, and appearance. The lycra fabrics are shiny while cotton blends are matte. You may prefer one over the other; cotton blends feel softer and more absorbent while lycra colors stay brilliant longer.

Dancewear has also gone beyond basic leotards and tights. The leotard itself may have long sleeves, short sleeves, or a tank appearance, and the leg holes may be cut high (the French cut). Tights may have "stirrup" feet or be footless, or end at the calf or even the knee. A unitard is a leotard and tights all in one, and while it is a struggle to get in and out of—and you may curse it when you need to go to the bathroom—nothing can beat it for feeling like a second skin, free of waistbands and leg elastic. There are tops and trunks, which are separate pieces that form a leotard. You can layer a tank leotard over a unitard, or trunks in a different color over tights. Many people find that layering different pieces gives you a variety of colors, looks, and a feeling of added support.

Finding a bra that fits can be a tremendous relief, as those of us with big breasts can attest. Bras designed specifically for running reduce the possibility of injury to breast tissue by distributing the weight more evenly and holding the breasts tighter to the chest wall, thus reducing bouncing. Their specially designed smooth seams reduce the potential for irritation created by regular bra seams and hooks. In the Appendix you will find listings of several running/ athletic bras in large sizes. Cotton or cotton blend next to your skin will be the most breathable and comfortable. You may have to try one or two to find the one that's most comfortable for you. It's worth the investment in a good bra to avoid back and shoulder pain as well as breast-bouncing discomfort. If you purchase a good bra and are still bothered by nipple irritation, try a bit of Vaseline on a cotton-reinforced pad (such as nursing mothers use).

If the Shoe Fits . . .

As you begin to know what you like to do the most, make appropriate shoes one of your first purchases. This means not only shoes that are designed for your particular activity but also shoes that fit your feet. There are hundreds of types of shoes. Shoe technology rivals NASA for sophistication as well as controversy, and there are more types being developed every day. We are not able to explore them all here, but we can give you certain basic principles to keep in mind when buying shoes:

1. Buy shoes. No, it is not a good idea to root around in the bottom of your closet, drag out your ten-year-old tennies, and go to an aerobics class or off on a hike over rocks and boulders, although a large woman in wedgies was spotted at the top of the three-mile, virtually straight-up switchback trail that leads to the top of Yosemite Falls. She was breathing hard and somewhat unsteady on her feet but, hey, she was there! It's just that she could have enjoyed it so much more in a pair of sturdy, comfortable shoes and avoided a great deal of discomfort on the following day.

    It's not even a great idea to use your old tennies for too many three-block walks to the store, although many women walk farther than that in high heels and live to tell about it. You could be lucky and not hurt yourself right away using your old shoes, and getting started in any shoes is to be respected. But even old tennies in perfect shape were just not built for aerobics or walking any distance, and they will not offer the kind of cushioning and support your feet, legs, and back need to avoid injuries and keep moving. When you begin to exercise more often, you may notice you want the shoes you wear around home to have good support too, particularly in the arch. Invest in your feet—they're the only ones you have.

2. Decide what activity you need shoes for, then buy and use them accordingly. Because most athletic shoes are relatively expensive, costing anywhere from $30 to nearly $100, you will probably want to use the shoes you buy only for the particular activity you are beginning. This is not only to save money by getting the longest wear out of the shoes but also to exercise safely. For instance, aerobics shoes are built to provide support for up-and-down movement in place. If you try to run out on a tennis court, where you need side-to-side stability, your shoes might not give you enough support. The same principle is true for running shoes, which are built for stability in forward motion but give little side-to-side stability. The planed sole sometimes catches during aerobics, making you more vulnerable to twisted ankles. Many people safely use running shoes for everyday walking, but for exercise walking, the new walking shoes offer better stability and support.

    The tread on the sole of the shoes also matters. Most of the new walking shoes, for instance, are not made for walking on steep hiking trails. You'll find yourself sliding downhill on your backside because the tread offers little traction. Sturdy running shoes or lightweight hiking boots with Vibram soles are better for traversing steeper, rocky terrain, and if you are carrying a heavy pack or contending with snow or water, you will want even heavier, ankle-high boots for support. All of these shoes should also have good arch support with uppers made of a material that breathes.

3. Buy from a knowledgeable salesperson. Usually this sort of person can be found in an athletic-shoe-only store, as opposed to a department store. If you want to be a more informed consumer, it's helpful to read up a bit on shoes ahead of time in the magazines or books that discuss your chosen sport or activity. Most athletic shoe stores now conduct special training sessions for their sales staff, and these salespeople should be able to tell you the difference between the types of shoes and which are appropriate for different activities. Of course, if the only pair of shoes they try to sell you is the most expensive one, think about shopping at another store. Just because it costs the most does not mean that it is automatically the right pair for you. There is a pair of $80 super-duper walking shoes sitting in one of the authors' closets at this very moment to attest to that.

    But most reputable stores will have sales staff who can look at your old shoes and watch you walk or run, and on that basis help you select a shoe that will give you the most stability and cushioning for the activity you want to try. They will also be able to show you shoes built specifically to reduce pronation (the tendency for feet to roll inward during movement) and supination (the opposite tendency, to carry the weight on the outside of the feet). They will be able to help you judge whether the width of the shoe fits both across the ball of the foot and the heel.

4.   Take your time, there's no rush. Take the socks you plan to wear and try on as many shoes as you need to find the ones right for you. Shoes should be comfortable right away; you should not need to break them in (with the exception of heavy hiking boots, for which your feet may need moleskin padding to prevent blisters). There should be at least a half inch between your big toe and the end of the shoe when your foot is in motion, so you may need an athletic shoe in a slightly bigger size than your street shoes. When you walk or twist to the side, your heel should not move around in the shoe. Lace-up shoes are of higher quality than the ones with Velcro closures, and offer a better fit, particularly if your heel is narrow.

If you have not had the pleasure of buying new, spiffy athletic shoes, it can be a wonderful treat. At a point when Pat was losing interest in running, a friend suggested getting a new pair of shoes to rekindle her former excitement. With a new pair she felt as though she was bouncing on air and ran right out of the store four miles down to the ocean. Another time when she was sidelined with a knee injury, a pair of aerobic shoes helped inspire her to dance at home. Shoes are definitely the "right piece of equipment" to help you get started or keep you going, and are usually worth the investment.

If you've never bought athletic shoes before and are wary of being intimidated by an overly jockish salesperson, take a friend with you for moral support. Most salespeople are there to make a sale rather than intimidate the customer. If you do run into someone rude, take your business elsewhere, as you would with any goods or services. Remember, it's your money. Once you have your new shoes, lace 'em up and off you go.

Finding a Class or Activity

We have listed in the Appendix all of the activities specifically for large women we know of as we go to press. We hope that many new ones have sprung up since then. If there are no activities listed in your area, that does not mean they aren't happening. For flyers or hot tips check with your local large-size clothing store, the local YMCA or YWCA, the Yellow Pages under "Exercise," and a few of the fitness studios in your area. Of course, you don't have to wait for an activity just for large women: try an ethnic dance class, yoga, T'ai Chi, etc. If these do not suffice, consider starting your own activity.

Starting an Exercise or Aerobics Class

The local Y or gym might be progressive enough to hire a teacher and start a class for large women based on your request, especially if you can show them a list of interested people ready to start coming. But if not, you can advertise and audition potential teachers yourself too. The power is in your hands, so use it! Decide before you propose the class to the Y or to a potential instructor exactly what you want and don't want:

About the Class. What should be the general purpose of the class? You need to decide this first, then find an instructor to reflect these principles. Personally, after years of being subjected to tirades about weight loss, I was sure I didn't want my We Dance class to stress weight loss; rather, we celebrate the joy of moving our bodies, sweating and playing hard together. You might prefer an instructor who is a large woman herself. You might want an instructor who has a background in dance or who obviously loves to dance. Or you may prefer someone with more fitness/exercise-oriented training. The teacher's training will have a big influence on whether you end up doing jazz dance movements or jumping jacks!

About the Students. Who are your fellow students? Should the class be restricted to women? Should the class be restricted to women of a certain size? If so, how big? You might open one class to any larger-than-average women and restrict one to women over two hundred pounds.

About the Activity.

- Do you want to include aerobic dance with your exercise? If so, require that it be nonimpact aerobics—that is, movements which challenge your cardio-respiratory system without jarring your joints and spine. Require that the pace be adjusted to the body size of the class members. Make sure the aerobics are fun for you.

- The class should be about an hour in length, including plenty of time to warm up and cool down your muscles at the beginning and end of the class, especially if you have an aerobic section. If the class consists only of calisthenics, make sure there is a balance between working a muscle and stretching it out. Your whole body should be exercised, with special attention to strengthening the abdominals (to protect the lower back) and the legs (to protect the knee joints) while maintaining proper alignment. You can use the We Dance exercises in this book to get started, or you can use those in Judy Alter's book, *Surviving Exercise* (see Appendix).

- What type of music inspires you to move? Make sure the instructor uses music that suits your tastes.

- Do you want the room you exercise in to have a mirror? Exercise mats? Lots of sunlight? Privacy from onlookers? Make sure your space has a floor that is wood, not concrete. Carpet over wood is okay but not carpet over concrete; the floor must have "give" to it to protect your joints and spine.

- Finally, suggest practical matters such as convenient times, number of times per week the class is offered, affordable price (perhaps a sliding scale if that is a need in your area), child care, and so forth.

About the Instructor.

- Assess the instructor's ability to move the class along smoothly, explaining necessary movements and positions without bogging down.

- In addition to style there is the issue of qualifications. Many schools now certify aerobics instructors. If the instructor has been certified by the International Dance-Exercise Association (IDEA), The Aerobic Fitness Association of America (AFAA) or the American College of Sports Medicine, or holds a degree from an accredited university in exercise physiology or physical education, s/he probably has a greater-than-average understanding of exercise principles. But there are undoubtedly instructors with adequate training in dance and exercise who lack these certifications, as well as instructors with such certification who are not sensitive to the particular concerns of large people, reflecting yet another area of controversy in this young industry.

- Your instructor should know CPR (cardiopulmonary resuscitation) and, if possible, basic first aid.

◆ Your instructor should be willing to learn from you and other class members about how to adapt what s/he knows to teaching a class for larger, heavier bodies. Never hire a teacher who maintains that pain is desirable or necessary for fitness, or who gives you the feeling that s/he pities you or punishes you.

At last we are about to make the transition from talking about exercise to doing it. The next chapter contains very important information about warming up, cooling down, and stretching. It's finally time to get your body involved!

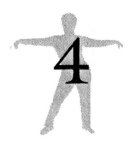

4

Warm-ups, Cool-downs, and Stretches

Imagine that you are standing on the banks of a beautiful, sparkling clear lake. First you put in your toe to test the water. Then you wade into the shallow water. You easily walk into the lake, and as the water becomes deeper, you smoothly glide into a swimming stroke. You feel your muscles gradually warming to the task, becoming more supple and strong. You begin swimming with all your power now, delighting in the feel of the water resisting your strong strokes. After a time you notice that you are nearing the opposite shore and that it is shallow enough to stand. You are breathing deeply as you switch to slow, easy steps toward the bank. As the water becomes shallower, it is easier to walk, and your breath returns to normal. On the soft, dry bank, you lay in the sun and languidly stretch your body, now flexible and sleek.

Doesn't that fantasy make your body purr? Your body likes to be treated gently, eased into and out of hard work, romanced a bit. No matter what kind of activity you decide to make the centerpiece of your exercise session, you need to warm up your muscles first and cool them down later.

During aerobic exercise your muscles contract, your blood pressure goes up, and your heart pumps a greater volume of blood to the working muscles. Gradually building the intensity protects your muscles and heart from sudden change, and tapering off allows your muscles to help pump the blood back to your heart as your blood pressure and heart rate slowly return to normal. Save your serious stretching for the end of your exercise session, after your heart rate has returned to normal but your muscles are still warm and supple. The muscles you worked have contracted in order to perform the exercise and need to be lengthened deliberately. That's also the time that stretching will feel the most satisfying to you.

How should you warm up? In general, for any given sport or activity, you can warm up by performing a slower, less intense version of the movements required by the activity. Simply going through the motions for a few minutes works. If you want more specific guidance, you can use the photos in this chapter. I have designed them to warm up the muscle groups we use in the We Dance program, which follows in Chapter 5.

Once you have warmed up, either by using these routines or by taking a few minutes to go through the motions of your activity, you're ready to play. You may want to build muscle strength and tone by using the exercises in the We Dance chapter or increase your cardiovascular fitness by performing the aerobic dance steps in that chapter. You may want to try walking or swimming, which are discussed in Chapter 6, or one of the other exciting sports discussed in Chapter 7. Whatever you decide, you will need to come back to this chapter for information on how to cool down and stretch after your activity.

Cooling down is just the reverse of warming up. Gradually lessening the intensity of your activity or simply walking around for a few minutes at the end helps bring your blood pressure and heart rate down gradually. The large muscles in your legs that have been flooded with blood during the aerobic phase help pump that blood back to your heart so it doesn't pool in your lower body. Once you are cooled down your body has returned to its resting state, but your muscles may still be tight.

That's where the stretching comes in. The general purpose of stretching is to lengthen muscles that have contracted to perform the work of exercise. Tight, constricted muscles are more vulnerable to tearing, and they will stay tight unless you stretch them afterwards. Have you ever noticed that when you make a tight fist and then relax your hand, your fingers stay curled up until you deliberately stretch them out? This is true of all your muscles. In everyday life some of our muscles are routinely stretched while others remain tight. Stretching out the tight, strong muscles (such as those in your lower back) and strengthening the loose, weaker muscles (such as your abdominal muscles) can help you move with more ease and power.

One cautionary note about how to stretch: Most of us have seen dancers or athletes "bouncing" as they stretch. They use the rebounding action to push themselves further into the stretch. This is called "ballistic stretching," and it is both unsafe and ineffective. Your muscles have a "stretch reflex," that is, they contract when they are yanked suddenly. If the overall purpose is to lengthen the muscle, it is important not to engage this reflex. Lengthening the muscle requires a long, slow, smooth movement. Breathe into the movement as you stretch. You will feel a natural limit in your range of motion, and that is the moment to relax. Forcing yourself past that position or into pain will make you stiff and sore.

The following pictures present only a very basic routine. You can consult several good books listed in the Appendix for more detailed stretching routines or stretches that are particularly good for the activity of your choice.

Here is how to use the pictures: Set A photos can be used as an initial warm-up or as a final stretch, depending on how you do the movements. To begin your exercise session, do a few rhythmic repetitions of each exercise simply to prepare your body for more strenuous work. Then go on to the Set B photos. Those movements are a little more lively and can serve as a transition to your main activity. You will have warmed up your body by going through these basic movements and can go ahead and do your main activity.

When you are ready to cool down, you can return to the movements in Set B as transition steps or simply walk around for a few minutes. The important thing is to taper off the intensity while keeping your legs moving. For a final stretch go back to the Set A photos, and this time work through them slowly and deliberately, relaxing into each position for at least 15 seconds. This more intense stretching is an excellent way to increase flexibility in the muscles you've "pumped" during your workout.

To recap: Make sure you warm up and cool down and make sure you stretch out at the end, not by bouncing but by slowly relaxing in the pictured position. Start with Set A and Set B to warm up, then do your main activity, then come back to Set B, and end with Set A.

Set A

If you are doing this set at the beginning of your exercise session, repeat each movement several times rhythmically. This warms up your muscles gradually. Conversely, if you are doing this set as a stretch at the end of your session, assume each position only once or twice, and relax into it longer, a good 15 or 20 seconds if possible.

Starting Position (front and side views)
Plant your feet a little wider apart than shoulder width. Soften your knees and let your tailbone relax. Unlike what you do in ballet class, you want to maintain the natural curve of your lower back. Take a nice big breath, and as you exhale, let your ribs stay lifted and your shoulders relaxed.

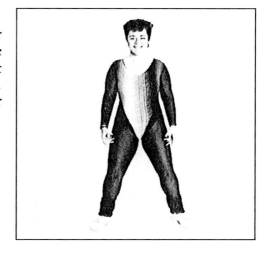

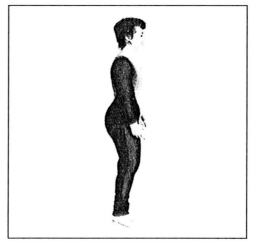

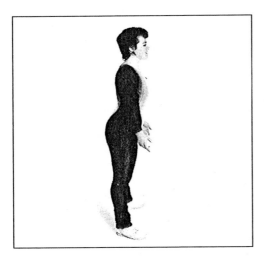

Wrong position #1: I've let my knees lock and my back arch.

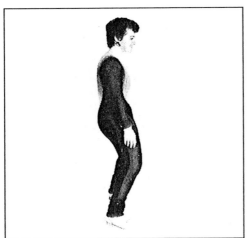

Wrong position #2: I'm trying to tuck my pelvis under (let the ballet dancers worry about that), and I've let my ribs collapse and my chin jut forward.

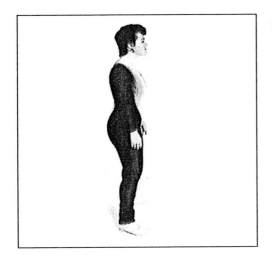

For Your Neck

Maintaining your starting stance, reach forward with your chin.

Then pull it straight back.

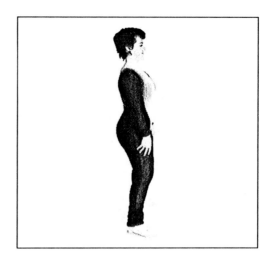

Drop your head forward. (Tilting the head back is not recommended. It is the back of the neck that needs stretching.)

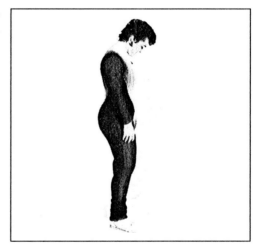

Tilt your ear toward your shoulder, letting your shoulders stay relaxed. Do the same on the other side.

Now let your head roll forward slowly from that tilted position through the forward position and to the opposite side tilt. You have just described a semicircle—half of a "neck roll," the half across the front of your chest. Reverse the path, again rolling your head only across the front of your chest.

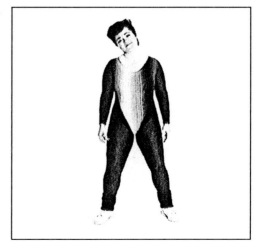

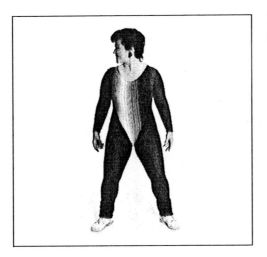

Look back over your shoulder. Do the same on the other side.

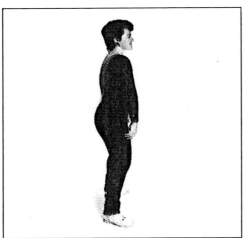

For Your Shoulders

Round your shoulders forward.

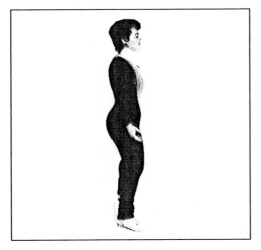

Pulling your shoulder blades together, stretch your shoulders back.

Lift your shoulders high.

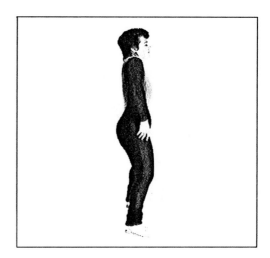

And push them down.

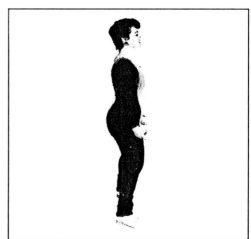

Shoulder Rolls
Roll your shoulders forward through each of these positions: up, forward, down, and back. Then reverse: up, back, down, and forward.

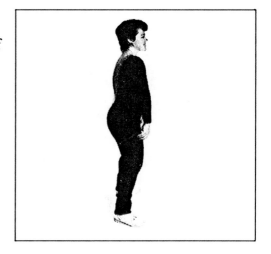

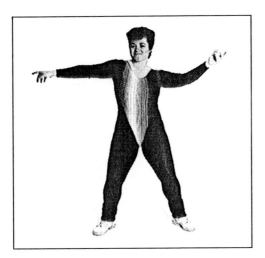

Shimmy Stretch
Push one shoulder forward, one back, arms lifted gently to the sides.

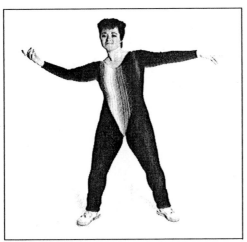

And shift. Repeat.

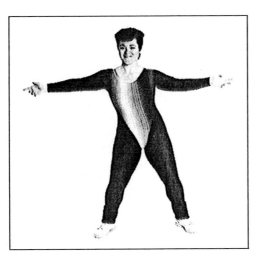

For Your Torso

Rib Cage Isolations
Leaving hips stationary, slide rib cage to left, letting shoulders follow and be relaxed.

Slide rib cage to the right. Again, allow shoulders to stay relaxed. Repeat movement left and right.

Notice that you don't tilt your shoulders in this exercise. Your rib cage and your hips are sliding past each other in opposite directions, both staying horizontal.

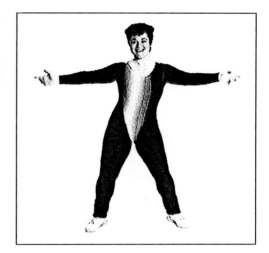

Check to see that your knees are still slightly bent. Reach the rib cage forward, letting everything else stretch back.

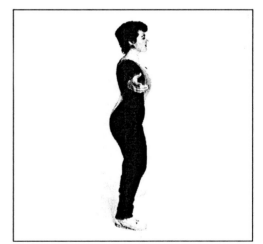

Now bring your rib cage straight back, allowing your shoulder blades to round out. Repeat movement forward and back.

Rib Cage Circles

For more of a challenge as you get to know the four positions for your rib cage (out and back, left and right), try moving just your rib cage around in a circle, beginning clockwise, then reversing to counterclockwise. Again, your hips stay stable.

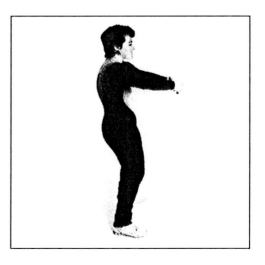

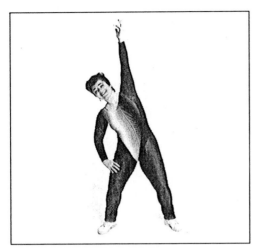

Waist Stretch

Bend the knees a little more and use one hand on the same-side thigh for support. Reach the other hand up and feel yourself lift your rib cage up and away from your hip. This is a way to stretch your side without putting undue pressure on your lower back. Do the same thing on the other side. Remember, lift your rib cage rather than your shoulder.

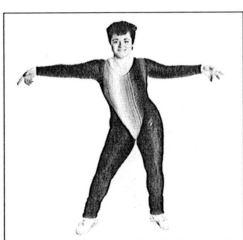

For Your Hips

Hip Isolations

Open your arms and swing your hips to the right. Then to the left.

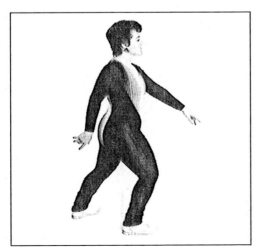

Placing one foot forward, shift your weight onto the forward leg, leading with your hips. You should feel a stretch in the inner, upper area of the other thigh as you push your pelvis forward.

Pull your hips back to shift your weight to the rear leg. As your pelvis becomes more mobile, you can "lead" with it more easily.

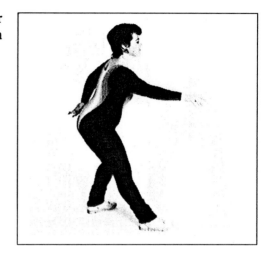

For Your Heels, Calves, and Hamstrings

Back of the Leg Wall Stretch
Bring your feet parallel (that is, toes pointing straight ahead) and slide one foot back. Place your hands against the wall.

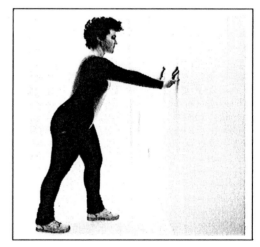

Bring your hips closer to the wall by bending the front leg. Keep the back heel down so that you feel the stretch in the back of your heel and the calf muscle. Make sure your back knee is not locked or hyperextended (that is, bend it slightly).

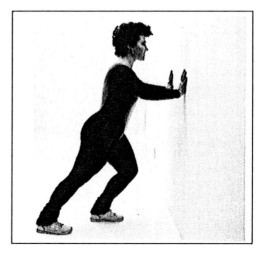

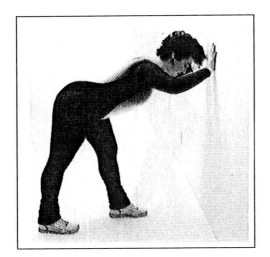

Now, using your hands against the wall for stability, lift your hips up to stretch the front leg. You should feel the stretch in the back of the thigh (the hamstring). Again, make sure you are bending both knees ever so slightly in order to keep from locking your joints or hyperextending. Reverse your feet and repeat on the other side.

If you would like to continue this set on the floor, the movements below give additional attention to your lower back, hamstrings, and abdominal muscles.

Most people spontaneously lower themselves to the floor in the most comfortable way. The important thing to remember is to use the strong muscles in your thighs and buttocks to lower yourself, rather than your back. A good method for many people is to place the legs wide open, bend the knees, lean forward, place both hands on your thighs (or, if you are flexible, on the floor), lower one knee to the floor, and lower your hips to the side to sit.

If you need help, ask! Someone can give you a hand, or you can use the support of a stable object such as the back of a sofa if you're at home or a fixed ballet barre if you're in a studio.

Make sure you have your exercise mat or some kind of padding within reach, as well as a towel, so you don't have to get up and down again.

Lower Back and Buttocks Stretch: Pull the backs of your knees toward you gently, letting them open if that's more comfortable, to release the lower back and buttock muscles.

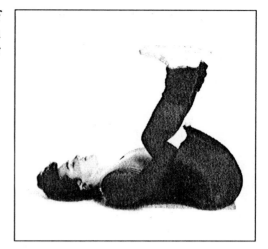

Hamstring Stretch

Place a towel just above the back of the knee, straighten your leg, then slightly bend your knee. Keep your knee slightly bent—not locked or very bent—as you gently pull the towel toward you. Pull only to the point where you meet resistance, then gently stay there for a few seconds.

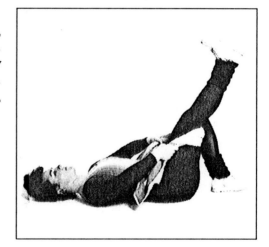

As you become more flexible you will be able to draw your leg closer. For more of a challenge, flex your foot. After stretching, do the same for the other leg.

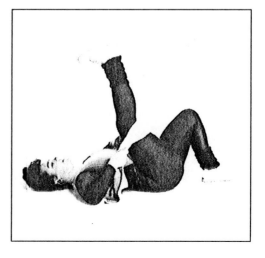

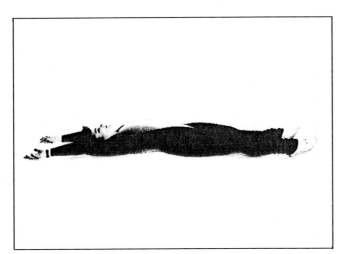

All-Body Stretch
To stretch out your stomach muscles, bring your legs straight and raise your arms overhead. From the tips of your fingers to the tips of your toes, make yourself as long as you can.

One method of getting up off the floor is pictured on page 90. Another is simply to reverse what you did to lower yourself to the floor. First roll to your side, drawing your knees in, and use your hands to push your upper body into a sitting position. From sitting, lift your hips so you're standing on your knees. Then place one foot in front of you and your hand on that thigh, and leaning forward, push off with the other leg to stand. As with getting on the floor, if you need help, you can ask a friend or use a stable piece of furniture to brace you.

End your stretch with a full, wonderful breath.

Exhale through your mouth to empty your lungs.

Inhale through your nose slowly, letting your breath fill you. Slowly exhale through your mouth. Repeat two more times.

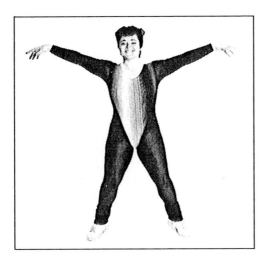

Set B: Transition Steps

Once you have completed the movements pictured in Set A, you might want a slightly more vigorous warm-up before you move on to your aerobic activity. Conversely, if you have completed your aerobic activity and need to bring your heart rate down gradually, you can use these movements to cool down.

Let yourself relax and get into the rhythm of the following movements, doing each one for a couple of minutes.

Knee Swings

Let one knee swing up, then the other. This is not a yanking motion; you are not trying to "get your knee to your chest" but rather enjoying the feel of swinging your legs.

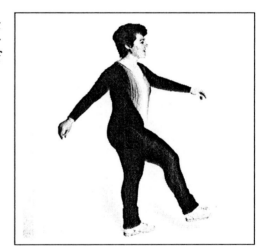

This is the same idea, but here you swing your leg open to the side, then swing out the other leg. Let your arms swing too.

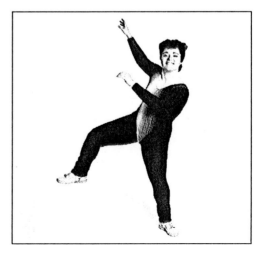

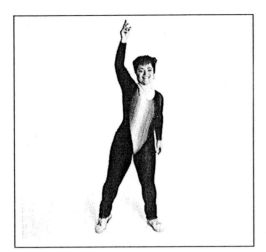

Reaching Up
On one, you reach with the same arm and leg;

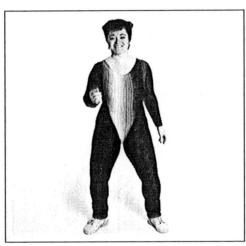

On two, you bring them both back in. On three, you reach with the other arm and leg, and on four, you bring them both back in.

You should feel pleasantly warm and supple at this point, ready either to intensify your warm-up in preparation for aerobic activity or to begin stretching out the muscles you already worked by going back through Set A.

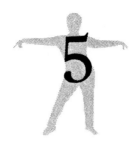

We Dance Exercises and Dance Steps

So you're all warmed up and ready to work and play.

The pictures on the following pages show some of what we do in a typical We Dance class: strengthening and stretching exercises, and aerobic dance. You can use just the exercise pictures, if you like, or just the dance steps, or you can do them both. Just make sure to sandwich the activities in this chapter with the warm-ups, cool-downs, and stretches in Chapter 4.

Tips About the Exercise Section

What's the goal of doing exercises? Well, it is not to reduce overall body fat because only an aerobic activity uses fat for fuel. Doing calisthenics is usually not challenging enough to boost the heart rate into the aerobic range nor is it consistent enough exertion to keep it there. And neither is the goal to "spot-reduce." Check the arms of your local tennis jock: If spot-reducing worked, her serving arm would be leaner than the other one. It might well be more muscular and more toned, but it is not leaner. Then why do exercises?

Judy Alter points out in her book, *Surviving Exercise,* that some of our muscles get stretched and loose from our daily routine while others become tight and strong. Using your exercise session to compensate for this can lead to greater ease and comfort when you move. You will notice, for example, that we do several exercises to strengthen the abdominal muscles, which are typically loose and weak from our daily activities, and we stretch the lower back and buttocks, which are typically tight. Balancing the strength of opposing muscle groups and increasing their flexibility will leave you feeling stronger and more graceful.

A second goal of these exercises is to strengthen and tone particular muscle groups. To do this it is very important that you maintain the proper alignment. If you allow your position to get wobbly during the movement, you will be using other muscle groups to help do the work, which sabotages your efforts to get stronger. This is why exercise instructors and dancers talk about "isolating" particular muscle groups. It simply means you hold the rest of your body steady so that the muscles you are focusing on can do the work.

Trying to make the movement overly big or fast also compromises your efforts to build strength. Many exercisers unthinkingly use momentum in their routines, yanking their body parts around to the beat. The phase of the exercise in which the muscle is building strength is the time that you are in controlled motion. Make your movements small, deliberate, and sustained. This will also protect your joints. As your strength grows you will be able to maintain your alignment and control within an increasingly wide range of motion.

How many repetitions should you do? Let your body decide. That burning sensation after you've done many repetitions of the same movement is lactic acid, a waste product, building up in your muscles. While "the burn" is not a sign of danger, shaking it out takes only a second or two and makes exercising more comfortable and less likely to make you sore the following day. You can use your own body to determine the proper number of repetitions by working, shaking out and working a little more, then shaking out a second time. You are using the burn to set a limit for you, rather than "going for the burn" itself.

Remember that differences in upper back and shoulder flexibility and chest endowment determine how close your elbows can pull together. The point is not to touch elbows but to work against your own limit. Limits in our range of motion provide a natural "resistance," and resistance, whether range of motion or weights, is what you need to build strength. This exercise builds strength in your chest wall muscles as well as flexibility across your upper back.

Wall Push-ups
A less challenging modification of push-ups. Begin with your feet at a comfortable distance from the wall, about shoulder width apart, and hold your torso steady.

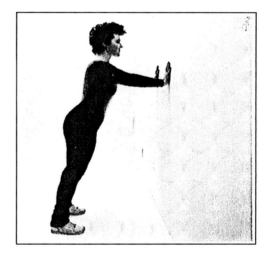

Bend at the elbows to lower your body toward the wall. Simply let yourself down slowly, say for a count of 8. If you need more of a challenge, lower your body, then push back up. At first make your push-ups shallow. As you build strength, deepen them; and when you can do them easily, move to the floor (see page 84).

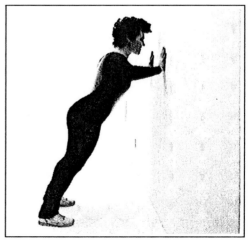

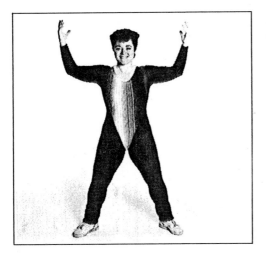

Pectoral Strengthener: Begin with arms in "touchdown" position, knees slightly bent.

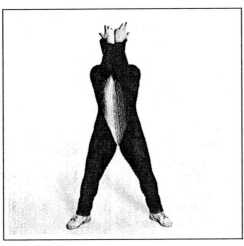

Keeping elbows as high as you can throughout, pull your elbows as close as possible, then open them to the starting position again.

Bicep Strengthener: After shaking your arms out, pull your elbows close again. This time, lift your elbows even higher while keeping them close, then let them lower. Shake your arms out if you feel your muscles burning.

Now we move to exercises done on the floor. Make sure you have a mat or a towel within reach.

A reminder about breathing as we begin the abdominal exercises:

Many people simply stop breathing while they're doing sit-ups or abdominal exercises. Don't! Here's how to time your breaths: On the exertion phase of the exercise (the *up* in a sit-up) you *exhale.* On the relaxation phase, you *inhale.* This is useful for any sort of exercise where you notice yourself holding your breath.

Lower Abdominals

Lie on your back, knees bent, feet flat on the floor, and hands cradling your head.

Press your lower back into the floor. You want to press the back of your waist hard against the floor, which tilts your pelvis slightly. This is the exertion phase, so you exhale. In fact, it will feel as if you are pushing the air out of your lungs. As you release your muscles, breathe in. Repeat.

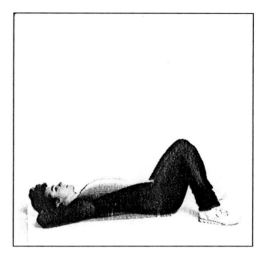

Curl-ups

Take one hand and rest it across your stomach, supporting your head with the other hand.

While pushing your lower back into the mat, curl your upper body forward. You shouldn't be able to sit up all the way. This is the exertion phase, so you breathe out. As you gently lower your upper body to the floor, breathe in. Repeat.

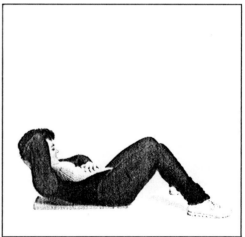

Diagonal Curl-ups

Cross the leg opposite the arm supporting your head.

Roll up so that you aim your armpit at the opposite knee. This is the exertion phase, so you breathe out. Notice that you are not trying to touch your elbow to your knee or otherwise crunch yourself up. Slowly release and breathe in. Repeat on the same side, then change to the other side.

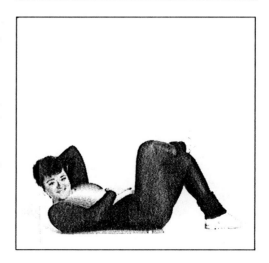

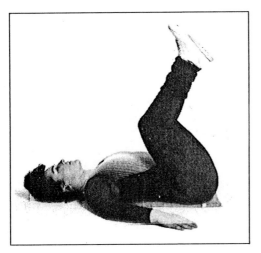

Knee Presses

For more of a challenge, place your arms out to the sides and bring your feet up. This exercise requires flexibility in your hamstrings, the muscles that run down the backs of your legs. In the rest position your knees can be open, but your feet need to be in line with your hips. If, as you see yourself from the side, your knees or feet are hanging out over empty space, don't do this exercise yet because you could hurt your lower back. But if you can rest with them at a right angle to your body, you can proceed.

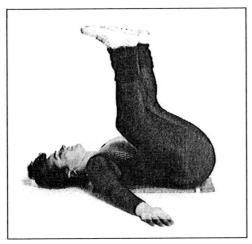

Pressing your lower back into the floor, draw your knees closer to your chest. This is the exertion phase, so you breathe out. Then release to the rest position as you breathe in. Remember, even at rest your legs should be at a right angle to your body. Repeat.

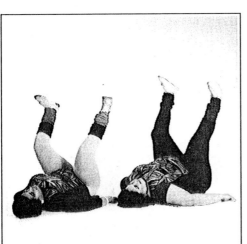

Rosemary and Frances show the correct alignment for this exercise. Knees over hips and lower abdominals pressing into the floor. You can let your knees open like this if it's more comfortable.

All-Body Stretch

To stretch out your abdominal muscles, lower your legs to the floor, straighten them, and raise your arms overhead. From the tips of your fingers to the tips of your toes, make yourself as long as you can!

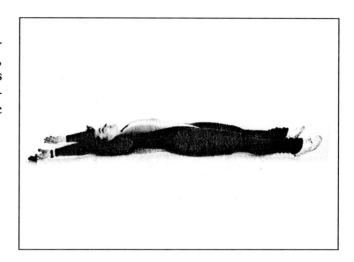

Buttocks Squeeze

Slightly lift your hips, then flatten the back of your waist against the floor. Hold in this position throughout. Squeeze your buttocks together and hold, then release.

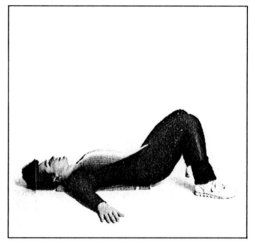

Lower Back and Buttocks Stretch

Pull the backs of your knees toward you gently, letting them open if that's more comfortable, to release the lower back and buttock muscles.

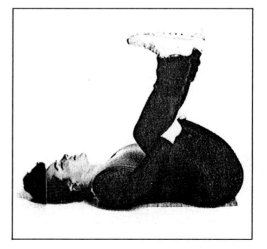

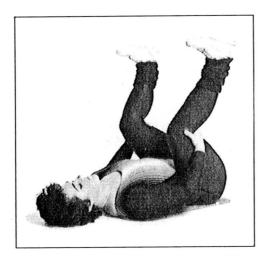

Foot Isolations
Holding the same position, flex your feet.

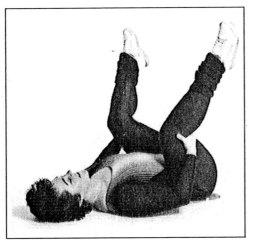

And point. Repeat. Then circle them clockwise and counterclockwise.

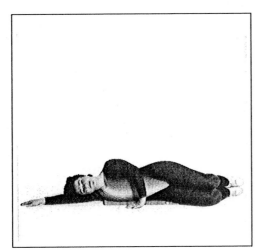

Outer Thigh Lifts
Begin on your side, head resting on your outstretched arm, other arm bracing you in front, hips and knees slightly bent.

Lift the top leg all of a piece. Notice that hips stay still, perpendicular to the floor, and the side of the thigh faces the ceiling throughout. If you find yourself twisting your leg around or dropping your hip back, start again and don't try to lift your leg so high. This is a small movement. The side of the thigh, not the front of the thigh, lifts the leg up. Release and repeat.

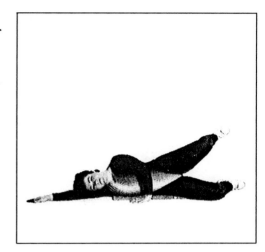

Inner Thigh Lifts

Draw your top leg up and forward, allowing it to relax on the floor in front of you, and extend the bottom leg.

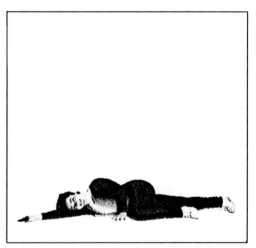

Flex the foot of your bottom leg, and keeping your knee straight, smoothly lift up from the inner thigh. This is a small movement. Release and repeat. When you have finished, swing your legs around and start with the outer thigh lift for your other leg.

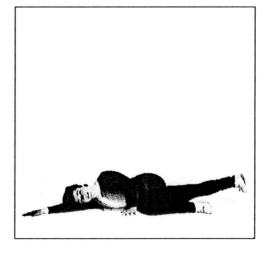

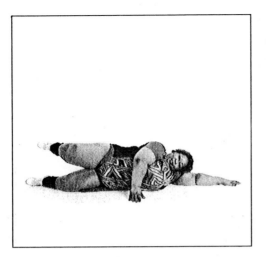

Peggy demonstrates the correct alignment for the outer thigh lift on the other side: The top knee stays lined up with the bottom knee, and her hip stays perpendicular to the floor rather than rocking backwards.

When you've finished with the outer and inner thigh lifts on the other side, smile, because *those* are over with for today!

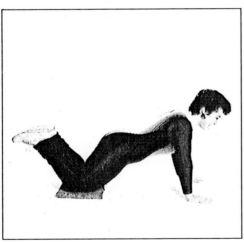

Bent Knee Push-ups

Roll over onto your stomach and place some padding below your knees. If you have graduated from wall push-ups, try these. The proper position for a push-up is to place your hands under your shoulders and hold your hips roughly in line with your knees and shoulders.

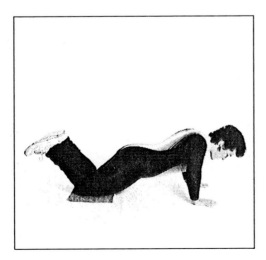

Letdowns

The first exercise to master is slowly letting yourself down, say on 8 counts. Don't let your hips sag or your back arch. Your torso stays all of a piece, and only your elbows move.

When you need more of a challenge, lower yourself and push back up. At first, don't lower yourself very far—maybe only half an inch! The point is not the distance but that you are working your arm muscles at their limit. Here Carol and Rosemary demonstrate the lowering phase.

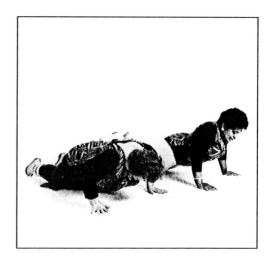

The triumph of mastering the push-up! As you need more of a challenge, lower and push back up increasing distances.

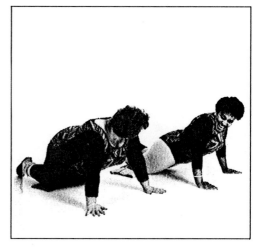

Positioning Yourself on All Fours
Make sure you put some padding under your knees. Your back is neither rounded nor swaybacked; maintain the natural arch throughout.

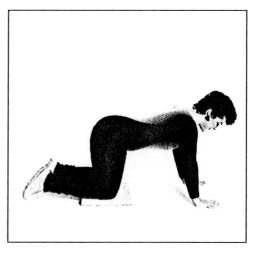

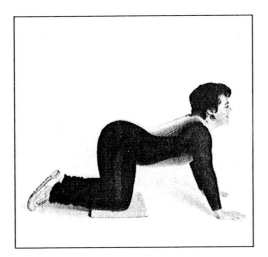

Wrong Position
As you do the following exercises make sure your back does not arch. Letting your back collapse like this puts undue stress on the lower back region.

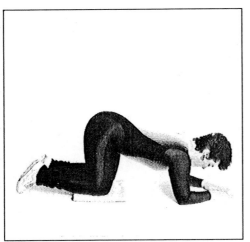

Lower yourself to your elbows, hands open.

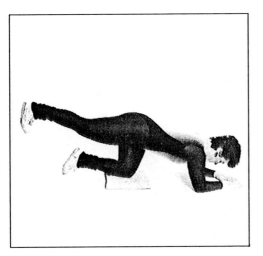

Extend your leg straight back.

Foot Pushes
Bend your knee and flex your foot. This is the start position.

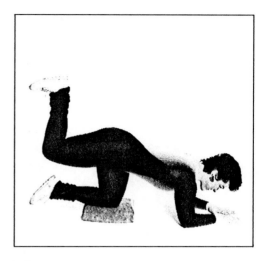

Push the bottom of your foot toward the ceiling. Notice that this is a small movement. Keep your hips square with the floor and isolate the movement in the back of your thigh and buttock. Let your knee slightly descend to the start position. Repeat.

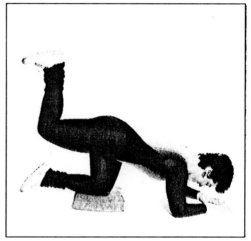

Wrong position
Notice I've let my hips open, and I'm completely off balance trying to get my leg too high.

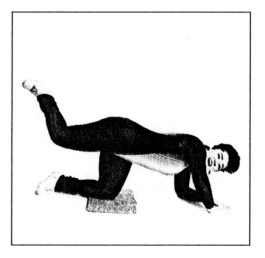

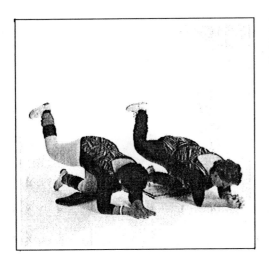

Rosemary and Robin demonstrate the correct position: hips are square with the floor, backs straight.

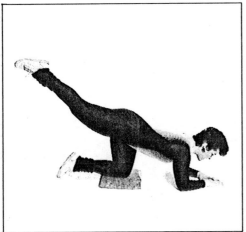

Leg Extensions
Before switching to the other leg, stretch your leg straight back, lifting it as much as you can without arching your back. Hold your thigh there.

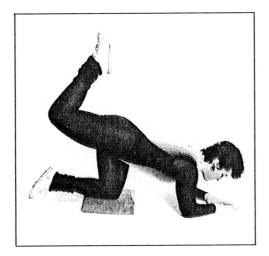

Bend your leg, then extend it. Repeat. Drop your knee and switch legs, starting with Foot Pushes.

Modifications for Sensitive Knees

If being on all fours is too painful for your knees, try lying on your stomach with padding under your hips and stomach. Bend your knee, flex your foot, and push the bottom of your foot toward the ceiling. Again, this is a very small movement that calls on the muscles in the back of your thigh and buttock rather than your lower back. Push and release.

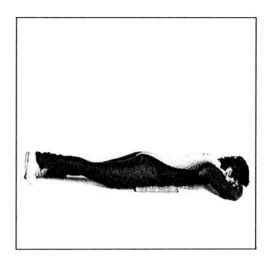

Modified Leg Extensions

Stretch your leg straight back, then bend and extend. Repeat. Change legs and begin with the above exercise using the other leg.

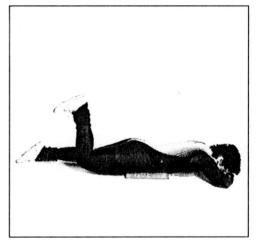

Buttocks Stretch

Push back onto your knees and let yourself sit a little to the side of your feet. Let the buttock and hip muscles stretch.

Shift your weight to the other side and stretch.

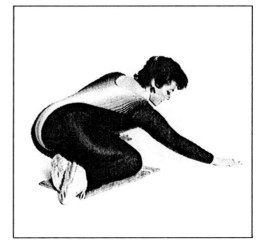

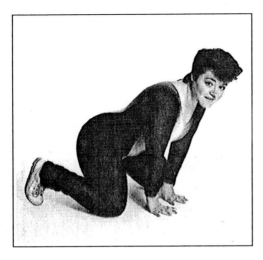

Pushing Up to Standing
Open your knees as far as you can and line your heels up behind them, tucking your toes under. Walk your hands in between your knees.

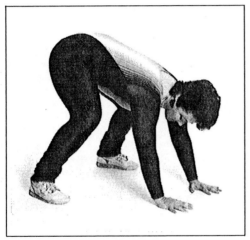

Push off from your hands, shifting your weight to your heels.

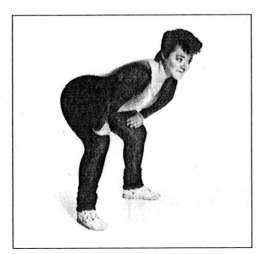

Shift your hands to your thighs.

Tip your body up to standing.

Half Squat

This last exercise strengthens your quadriceps (the big muscles on the front of your thighs) and buttocks. The image to hold in your mind is to simply sit yourself down, maintaining the natural curve of your back.

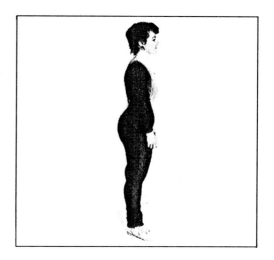

Use your hands on your thighs for support as you bend your knees and sit.

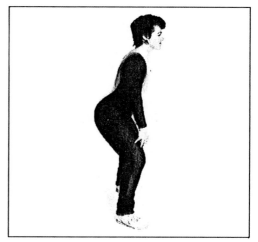

Don't go any lower than this. When your thighs are almost parallel to the floor, reverse the process and stand up. Repeat.

Shake everything out before you begin your aerobic session, including your head, shoulders, arms, ribs, hips, buttocks, thighs, feet, and hands.

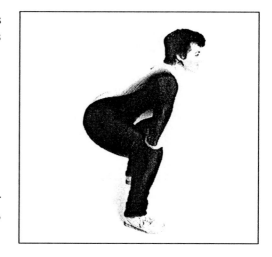

Now that you have completed the strengthening exercises, you can either stretch out those muscles you've been working or postpone stretching until after you've danced or done another kind of aerobic activity. To stretch now, go back to Chapter 4 and do Set A. To continue with an aerobic activity, read on to find out about taking your pulse, and then you can either use the dance steps pictured or do the aerobic activity of your choice. Afterwards, remember to cool down gradually by slowly tapering off your activity or by using the movements in Set B. And remember to stretch using Set A.

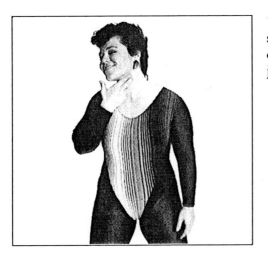

Taking Your Pulse: Before you begin the aerobic session, locate your pulse. One location is your carotid artery, just to the side of your throat and just under the jaw.

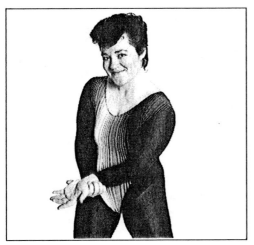

The other location is your wrist, on the inside. Use the first two fingers rather than your thumb (which has a strong pulse of its own).

Locating your pulse takes practice, and it is easier when your heart rate increases, as it does when you're exercising hard. Take your pulse midway through your aerobic session and compare it to your target rate (see Finding Your Target Heart Rate, page 42). If your actual heart rate is lower than your target, you can afford to get more rambunctious! If it is higher, don't stop completely but ease up a bit, then take your pulse again in a few minutes. In this way you can adjust your exertion level to maintain your target heart rate.

How long should you keep up your aerobic activity?

Start with a brief period (5 minutes) and stay at the lower end of the target zone (65 percent of your maximum heart rate). You should stay at 65 percent as you gradually increase your time; and when you've worked up to 20 minutes, you can move your target to 70 percent of maximum. Beyond 85 percent of maximum is the point of diminishing returns, so that's your outer limit. Ultimately, 20 to 35 minutes of aerobic activity, three times a week, is enough to maintain your fitness level. If you find one or more activities that delight you and make time in your life for them, you may be surprised one of these days to realize you're maintaining that three-times-a-week schedule with little effort and much enthusiasm.

We Dance Steps

If a picture is worth a thousand words, a video is worth a thousand pictures. But while we are waiting for the We Dance video (still a gleam in this author's eye), photographs will have to do.

Each of the pictured steps runs in a 4- or 8-count cycle. Most popular music is compatible with this rhythm. Turn on the radio or put on a song you like, music that makes you feel like tapping your toe.

How long should you do each step? As long as you like. At first you need to spend time going slower and learning the moves. Then after you get used to the steps, you can go from one to another, changing after you get tired of one or changing because the musical phrase in your song changes. The advantage of using a book rather than a video or class is that you can dance according to your own whims.

	COUNT	SAY
The Charleston		
Step out on your right foot	1	*Step*

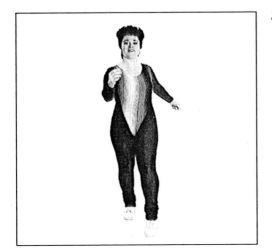

Swing your left foot up past it	2	*Touch*

Step back on your left foot   3   *Step*

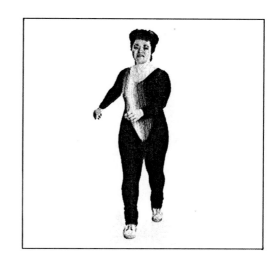

Swing your right foot back past it.   4   *Touch*

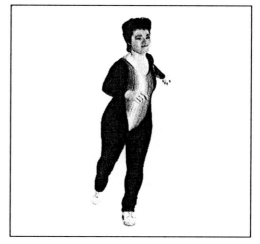

Once you've got that, try it starting with the left foot.

If you want to try something really advanced, practice going smoothly from one side to the other.

Transition to the Other Foot

It's almost the same but you change the last beat:

	COUNT	SAY
Step out on your right foot	1	*Step*
Swing your left foot up past it	2	*Touch*
Step back on your left foot	3	*Step*
Step back on your right foot	4	*Step*
Step out on your left foot	5	*Step*
Swing your right foot up past it	6	*Touch*
Step back on your right foot	7	*Step*
Swing your left foot back past it.	8	*Touch*

See? You're on the other side now. Practice going back and forth!

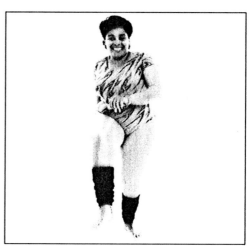

COUNT   SAY

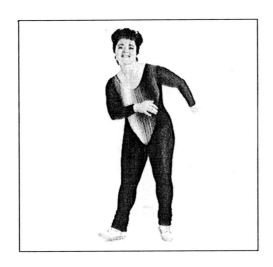

The Stroll
Step out to the side with right
foot   1   *Step*

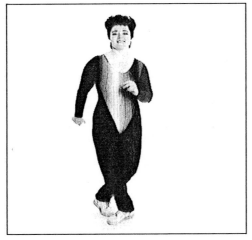

Cross your left foot behind the
right   2   *Cross*

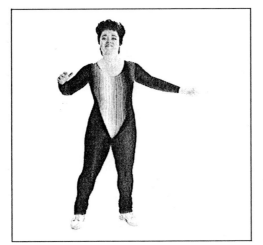

Step out again with your right
foot   3   *Step*

Draw your left foot into your
right, ready to reverse: 4   *Touch*

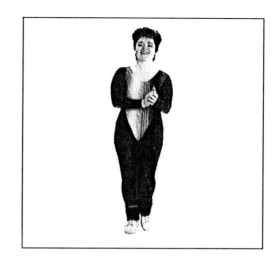

Step out to the side with your left
foot   5   *Step*
Cross your right foot behind the
left   6   *Cross*
Step out again with your left foot   7   *Step*
Draw your right foot in, ready to
start over.   8   *Touch*

COUNT   SAY

Box Step
Step forward with your right foot   1   *Step*

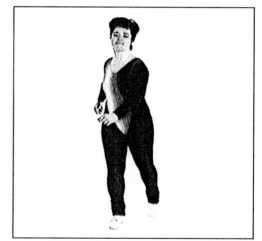

Cross your left foot way over your
right and lean forward   2   *Cross*

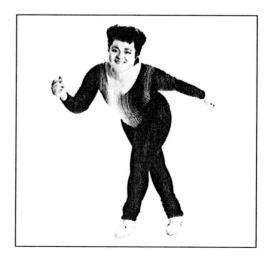

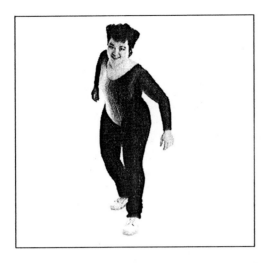

Roll your weight back to your left
heel, pushing off the front foot to
step back onto your right one   3   *Shift*

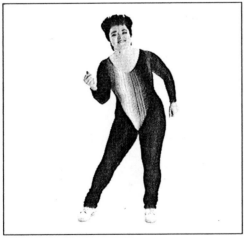

Draw back and step on your left
foot, ready to start over.   4   *Step*

Once you've got the rolling motion of this step,
try it starting with your left foot forward.

There are many other informal dance steps that you can use in your routine. Step out to the side on the right foot, then draw the left foot in to touch; step out to the side with the left foot, then draw the right foot in to touch. This "step-touch, step-touch" step is very basic and can be combined with others. For example, do the stroll to the right, then step-touch, step-touch; then take the stroll to the left, and step-touch, step-touch.

The Rocking Step is on the same basic pattern as "step-touch, step-touch":

	COUNT	SAY
Step onto your right foot and lean forward	1	*Step*
Bring your back foot in to touch and snap your fingers	2	*Touch*
Step back on your left foot	3	*Step*
Draw your right foot back to touch and snap your fingers, ready to start again	4	*Touch*
Try it starting with your left foot first.		

Don't forget to pepper your routine with such things as side-to-side hips, reaching alternate arms, and so forth. You can march, skip, gallop, twist, pony, swing your knees up, and so on, to the music. To make your movements low impact, always keep one foot on the floor; it is when you land with both feet in a jump or hop that your legs experience higher impact, and the risk of injury increases. So, as Ann Landers says, "Keep one foot on the floor!" and as I say, "Everybody paaarrr-ty!"

When you're finished dancing, cool down by walking around continuously for a few minutes. This is as important as warming up. Remember, after aerobic exercise your blood pressure is raised, and there is a greater volume of blood in your large muscle groups, that is, your legs. Walking around uses your leg muscles, which helps pump the blood back up to your heart. Your blood pressure can descend gradually.

When your breath has returned to normal, take your pulse. It should be under 120 beats per minute, and ideally under 100, before you stop walking and start stretching. If you have led a sedentary life recently, it will take longer for your heart rate to return to its resting pace. As you condition your heart over time, you will notice that your pulse recovers more quickly and that you need more of a physical challenge, more exertion, to boost it into the target range in the first place.

Once your pulse has dropped and your breathing has returned to normal, go back to the stretching exercises (Set A in Chapter 4). Your now-warm muscles are more flexible and can comfortably stretch further. Also, they are contracted from doing the physical work of calisthenics and dancing and need to be lengthened. Muscles don't relax by themselves—they need to be stretched, either deliberately or incidentally through your daily activities.

Use the pictures in Chapter 4 as a guide. The goal is not to "get into" the pictured position but to stretch in *that direction*. Different people have different flexibilities. You are trying to lengthen the muscle rather than the tendons (which attach the muscle to the bone) or ligaments (which hold your joints together). Tendons and ligaments, when stretched, don't snap back. That is why it is important not to overbend or hyperextend a joint.

To stretch a muscle you must relax and breathe and let it release. Each stretch takes 20 to 30 seconds. This can be a very enjoyable part of your exercise, and it leaves you feeling, like the Tin Man, oiled and polished!

Once you have stretched, take a moment to thank yourself for taking the time to move and play. Treat yourself to a luxurious bath or a massage to prolong the pleasure. And think about when you can set aside the time to do it again!

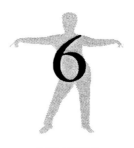

6

I'd Walk a Mile for a Swim

Walking and Swimming for No Pain, All Gain

Walking and swimming are two of the most popular fitness activities around because they are familiar, accessible to most people, pleasurable, as challenging as you want them to be, and very low risk. They can be done individually or with others, and indoors or outside depending on the season; they are as close as your front door or neighborhood pool. You can do them interchangeably, to offer variety in your week's activities, or you can get totally enraptured with one or the other. Check them out and then decide if they are for you.

One Foot in Front of the Other

Meet the Oakland Raters

Alice and Cheron started going for walks as a way to both spend time together amid hectic schedules and to get some exercise. To add a little spice, they turned each walk into a mini-adventure. "We laughingly began calling ourselves the Oakland Raters because we'd pick a different neighborhood for each walk and then rate them as we went—landscaping, paint jobs, the best looking or the tackiest houses on the block, things like that. We'd have a few great laughs and get our exercise at the same time.

"Lately, though, we've begun going to a local park that has dirt trails covered with pine needles because walking on them is so much softer than walking on cement," continued Alice. "It seemed as though my body was beginning to ache constantly—my legs, feet, and back began crying for relief. Now, since we're not walking on cement all the time and since I also bought a pair of shoes with lots of cushion and support, my body feels fine. No more aches! Just the fun of walking, breathing lots of fresh air, and checking out the scenery along the way. I love it and look forward to it. I'd really miss it if we stopped."

Now these folks have the right idea. A little togetherness for motivation and camaraderie, a spirit of fun and inventiveness to keep things interesting, enough attention given to business to adjust the activity to what your body needs and, presto, a form of exercise that you can look forward to! Not punishment but enjoyment. When you are considering what kind of exercise you want to try, it's important to keep these elements in mind. Most important in getting started is to look around you to see what's easiest and most accessible for you to do, then begin. Walking is one of the most accessible forms of exercise, one whose possibilities have been virtually overlooked until the last few years. Whether you start inside your house, in your yard, cruising around rating neighborhoods, or taking off on more adventurous trails, walking may be just the exercise ticket for you.

Walking is now one of the fastest growing fitness activities in the country, and in 1986 it even spawned its own slick magazine. Whether on city streets, country roads, beaches, or in parks, walkers seem to be everywhere. In some areas of the country where winter temperatures threaten even the hardiest enthusiasts, shopping malls have created special early-morning or late-day hours for walkers. With the right pair of cushioned shoes, walking is a no pain, all gain kind of activity, one that you can do regardless of where you live.

As with any new activity, start out slowly and gradually build up your muscle strength, heart and lung capacity, and endurance. You might begin by walking to do some errands and eventually build into your schedule a walk of 30 to 60 minutes, or even longer, several times a week. If you want to challenge yourself further, you may want to put a few hills into your route or perhaps take a longer hike on the weekend to explore the great outdoors. But remember, every walk begins with simply putting one foot in front of the other.

Don't Forget to Warm Up and Stretch

The importance of warming up and stretching, both for avoiding injury and gaining flexibility, cannot be overstated. No matter what form of exercise you choose, the warm-up and stretch should be a consistent part of your routine, as should the cool-down. Chapter 4 covers the idea of warm-up and the basic stretches you can do for a variety of activities, so if you began this chapter without reading that information, return to that section of the book in order to be well prepared for safe, injury-free exercise.

A complete aerobic walking routine could resemble the following plan: Begin by walking around your house for a few minutes to warm up. Warming up is just that simple—do your exercise but at a gentle, slow pace to let your heart and muscles gradually know they're going traveling. Next begin your walk at a slow pace and then gradually increase it until you reach your aerobic level. Exercise at your aerobic target heart rate for the amount of time you wish—at least 15 to 20 minutes is suggested by most fitness advisers—and then gradually decrease your pace until you want to stop. Coming to a gradual, not a sudden stop is your cool-down. Then you will want to go through a stretching routine when you arrive back home.

In deciding about your stretching routine, essentially you want to get a picture in your mind of the muscles you used during exercise and gently stretch them. Pay particular attention to the stretches for your legs and lower back. Spend several minutes with these. It's also important to rotate both ankles in clockwise and counterclockwise circles; point, flex, and relax the muscles in your feet; and go slowly up and down on the balls of your feet a few times. Since many of us carry tension in our neck and shoulders, which can increase during exercise if we're not aware of it, this is also a good time to do the gentle side-to-side stretches suggested for your neck and to rotate your shoulders in a circle forward a few times, and then reverse.

This complete cycle—warm-up, exercise, cool-down, stretch— is one that maximizes the overall fitness benefits of walking while it minimizes your chances for injury. And it is a complete routine that many people ignore. Too often both beginners and more experienced activity seekers ignore everything except the *exercise* phase and end up with an injury. If anything can discourage you in the first steps of a more active life, it is an injury. If you pay particular attention to each part of the exercise cycle, you will not be sidelined unnecessarily.

Now many times you may decide that you simply want to go out for a stroll and enjoy the evening breezes or catch the sunset, and you do not want this entire fitness cycle. In that instance you may be doing the warm-up phase throughout your walk; you may not actually increase your pace to an aerobic level, which is fine. Any walking, even getting off the bus a few stops before your usual one, aids you in achieving a goal of becoming more active and should be valued for itself. You may decide that stretching is not so important if you're just out strolling. However, even a few minutes spent stretching adds to your overall flexibility and eventually makes living in your body much more comfortable. Even after a slowly paced evening stroll, gentle stretching of warmed muscles upon your return home will enhance feelings of relaxation. The more you begin to associate any increase in activity with an accompanying increase in stretching, the more likely it is you will obtain more gain without pain. Here are a few more walking tips to help you get the most out of it.

Choose your surface.   As one of the Oakland Raters mentioned, the surface you walk on has a lot to do with how your body will feel overall. While some people can tolerate walking on cement sidewalks, others cannot. Cement or blacktop has no "give" whatsoever. Therefore, your body must absorb the impact of meeting this hard-as-a-rock surface with each step. If you notice that after the first few weeks of walking you still have aches and pains that are getting in your way or even making you want to quit, try changing the surface you are walking on. Better yet, start out on surfaces that give.

Be inventive! Virtually every town has some sort of park with dirt trails or grassy meadows, so use them. Walk on the grass strip next to the sidewalk or on boulevards. If you are lucky enough to live near a beach, you can try walking on the sand closest to the water line. This surface is firm enough so you don't feel as though you're plowing through the desert, but it has enough give to absorb the impact of your steps. Paying attention to the surface you walk on not only does your body a favor but your spirit as well. When you avoid cement and crowded intersections and look for grass or dirt you will probably find trees and flowers too. And as the old saying goes, we could all probably benefit by stopping more often to smell the flowers along the way.

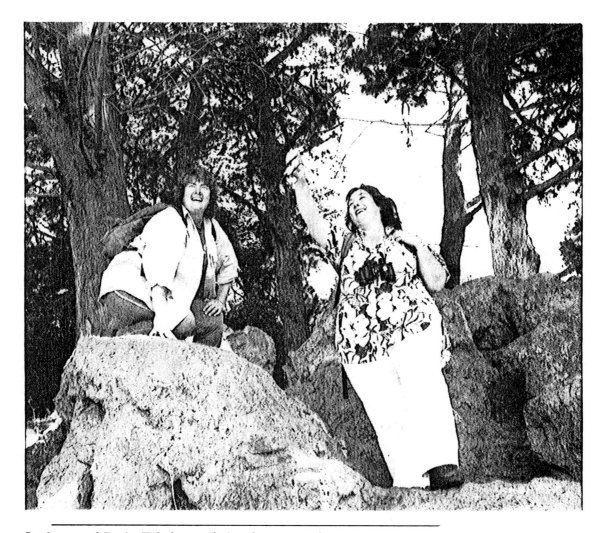

Pat Lyons and Danita Kulp love exploring the great outdoors.

Drink plenty of water before and after your walk. This is a rule of thumb for all exercise but particularly for aerobic exercise, which involves working up a sweat. The sweating is good for you, acting as your body's cooling system when evaporation occurs, but you need to replace the lost fluids. The best idea is to empty your bladder, have a large glass of water before you depart, and then drink some more when you're finished. While beer may taste great after exercise and has become the drink associated with sports, any alcohol eventually works to dehydrate you. Be sure to drink plenty of plain old tap water and don't add ice. Water that is too cold can be a shock to your system after exercise. If you get into long walks or hiking, carry water with you. You can't depend on streams to be clean enough to drink from, and you'll need water to keep going, particularly if you are climbing hills.

Pay attention to the weather.   Heed the advice offered by Charles Kuntzleman in his *Complete Book of Walking,* to avoid walking when the temperature reaches 85 and above, particularly if it is humid. In humid weather the body's cooling system is thrown off balance because sweat does not evaporate. If you sweat profusely while you're walking, your body can run out of water, resulting in a reduction in circulation, a drop in blood pressure and, eventually, heat exhaustion. To avoid this drink plenty of water, dress in light clothing, and avoid walking in the heat of the day. In summer months try walking in the very early morning or later in the evening when temperatures are cooler. Some enterprising city and suburban walkers use their local air-conditioned shopping mall.

Dress for success in cold weather by using layers.   Layers of clothing trap warm air between them, and this acts as additional insulation. When you start out on your walk you may be chilly, but once you get going you'll warm up and can then remove layers as you go. Try wearing breathable cotton next to your skin (or investigate more high-tech materials that wick moisture away from your skin without losing warmth), a sweat shirt or sweater, and a Windbreaker or jacket. If it's windy, a turtleneck or scarf is invaluable to keep your neck warm. Remember that heat escapes fastest through your head, so wearing a hat or cap is a good idea. Gloves also add a surprising amount of warmth, so you might be able to remove a heavier sweat shirt or jacket if you keep your gloves on. Experiment to find your comfort zone.

None of your walking gear needs to be fancy, mind you, but simply practical for starting out. On the other hand, buying clothes you like and wearing them just for walking can be a real incentive. Just as you may feel more like a business woman in a suit or like a dancer in a leotard, colorful sweats can make you feel more like a walker and add a positive spring to your step.

Prevent an age-old problem.   By putting Vaseline on your inner thighs you reduce chafing when wearing shorts but not when wearing a skirt (definitely too messy). Tights work pretty well to reduce friction under both shorts and skirts. Sweat pants probably work best of all, both to prevent chafing and to absorb the sweat that aggravates the problem. (Someday sweat pant makers may even learn to doubly reinforce the inner thigh, which wears out so fast. What a drag it is to have your favorite sweats be in perfect shape everywhere else but worn through in a month in the inner thigh area.)

Walk tall and proud. Not only is looking down at the ground likely to be more boring than looking at trees and people, but poor posture makes any walk more tiring. If you are bent over at the waist, particularly when walking up hills, the smooth circulation of oxygen through your bloodstream is reduced, and you will tire more easily. Try to keep your back straight and your shoulders down and back but relaxed, not stiff. Form an image in your mind of moving along effortlessly and smoothly even though you may be going very slowly.

Take the "talk test" while you walk. Earlier you learned to take both your resting and your aerobic target heart rate. Maintaining your pulse at your target rate will give you the most aerobic benefit from your walking. Walking faster than your proper rate is not only less enjoyable because you will be huffing and puffing, but it does not give you maximum benefit. You will end up tired, not refreshed, and you're more likely to quit as a result. If you are going at an aerobic pace that is right for you, you will be able to sing a song or maintain a conversation and not get out of breath. Regular, relaxed breathing is the goal, not huffing and puffing. If this means going very slowly, at what seems to you a turtle's pace, just remember that the turtle finished the race while the hare burned himself out. Better to start slowly, enjoying yourself, and keep at it for the long haul.

Some people find it helpful in the beginning to wear a watch and measure their pulse rate after about 10 minutes of walking to be sure they have reached but not exceeded their target heart rate. Eventually you will be able to tell when you are in your target zone simply by the way your body feels. After an initial period of warming up and gradually increasing your heart rate, it all of a sudden becomes easier to walk; usually it is at this point that your body has shifted into aerobic gear. Once your fitness level starts to improve you'll notice that walking at your proper aerobic pace often feels as though you could walk forever and not get tired. But it will take time for you to get to know your body well enough to tell when you have shifted into aerobic gear, so using a watch in the meantime is very helpful.

Arm swing.   If you've ever stuck your hands in your pockets and then tried to walk up a hill, you know how awkward it feels. A full, strong arm swing not only helps maintain balance and natural body rhythm but aids in distributing oxygen throughout the body by acting as a sort of pump. Thus, you can walk farther without tiring as quickly. On the other hand, too much arm swing can pick up your pace too much, and you will tire sooner. Fitness walkers who espouse a vigorous workout suggest bending your arms and imitating a soldier marching, but it's hard to imagine much relaxed enjoyment coming from marching around like a soldier. You may be limited in how much you can swing your arms if your upper arms are very large or if you carry a lot of weight on your upper body. A strong arm swing may not be possible without physical discomfort. No problem. The most important thing is to feel as comfortable as possible and not feel self-conscious by trying physically awkward movements. Concentrate on a smooth, even arm swing. You'll get to know how much is right for you after some experimentation.

Companionship versus time alone.   Walking with a partner is fun, and this is probably the only exercise you can do while holding hands. If you get your kids involved and they can keep up with your aerobic pace, you can forget about child care. But don't let your kids slow you down or distract you if your intention is to walk vigorously. A commitment to walking with another person can be just the thing to get you going when, left to your own devices, you might decide it's not so important today and skip it. This is particularly important during the first six weeks of your walking since it takes about that long to really get both your body and your schedule adjusted to the new routine.

On the other hand, solitary walking gives you a chance to soak up the beauty of the day without the distractions of conversation. As a stress reducer, particularly after a busy day of work, there's nothing quite like a brisk walk with some quiet time to yourself. It may, in fact, be the one time during your day when you are alone, offering you a chance to quiet your mind and simply enjoy your own company. This of course does not have to be a rigid, either-or choice but can vary with your needs so that you have both time alone and with friends.

Timing isn't everything.   But it can certainly make the difference between viewing exercise as a chore or as an enjoyable activity you look forward to. Some people love watching the sun come up, the quiet freshness of that part of the day. Others would find it torture to get up with the sun but love to walk at lunchtime as a refreshing break in a hectic day. To still others, a walk home from work is the perfect transition, enabling them to be fresh for family or friends, not bogged down in the day's events. And walking with a partner in the evening may be just the sleep aid you need, although if you wait until very late in the day you might feel too tired to get out there. You may know right away what time will work best, or you may need to experiment with different times. Just keep in mind that you are more likely to do your walk and enjoy it when the timing is right.

Pick a route you like. Some people love routine and want to walk the same route all the time. Others get bored by routine and want variety—a different neighborhood every day. People who like the feeling of going somewhere need a destination and might, for example, enjoy walking to or from work. Others are happy walking around a track, chalking up their numbers. Some people decide how much time they want to spend and then find a route that fits within this time frame, which allows them to build the walk into their regular schedule. Other people start out with a goal—one, three, five miles, for example—and will take whatever time is necessary to work toward that goal. Suit yourself.

The important thing is that you like the route you choose, that you make your exercise time a top priority in your schedule, that the goals you set are your own, and that you get satisfaction and enjoyment from your walking. With these tips in mind you can lace up your shoes and be off! Once you begin walking you'll realize how much more of the world you have access to. While once you may have gotten tired walking around the shopping mall or going up a short flight of steps, after a while you'll build up enough lung and leg power to go places you'd never dreamed possible.

One Very Realistic Fear

While walking offers a low chance for injury, it is not totally without risk, unfortunately. The daily newspaper is an all too vivid reminder of the dangers women face in the world. Harrowing attacks on women make safety precautions an absolute necessity these days.

One survey conducted by the North American Network of Women Runners found that "72 percent of respondents had experienced annoying comments, heckling or harassment; 59 percent experienced attempts by drivers to interfere with their running; 30

percent had feelings of being on display in a negative way; 5 percent had been assaulted. A full 81 percent reported that concern for the possibility of rape or harassment directly influenced when, where, or how often they ran." It is difficult to measure how much fear of violence or harassment directly affects women's freedom to exercise out in the world, but we believe the impact is considerable.

There is an extremely offensive myth that fat women don't get raped because they are not "sexually desirable." Rape is a crime of violence against women and has nothing to do with sexual desirability, body size, age, or any other such factor. This unfortunate reality was borne out in the experience of a Spokane, Washington, woman who despite two rapes continued to walk late at night alone in an effort to lose one hundred pounds. She said later that she was too embarrassed to walk during the daytime because she had to endure abuse and insults. When raped a third time she still did not report the attack immediately to the police because, as she said when she finally did go to the police, she thought "people would snicker because I'm fat. They would say he didn't rape me because I was repulsive."

It is an outrageous comment on our society that some women feel it is better to risk (or even worse, endure) rape in the dark than to walk in the daylight world as larger women. It is also sad but true that rapists also attack us in broad daylight and in the presumed security of our own homes. So until men stop their violence against women, we must acknowledge the risks and take steps to protect ourselves. Solitary night walking is never a good idea, particularly in urban areas. Choose well-lighted, well-populated routes or, if walking in less populated or unfamiliar areas, go with a partner or take a dog with you. If you go to an unfamiliar part of town for a class, be sure you have specific directions and ask about parking. Keep your keys handy to get back in your car or house quickly. Trust your instincts. If someone looks or acts suspiciously or if you sense you are unsafe, *act,* don't ignore your instincts. Yell *Fire!*—not help— because more people will pay attention. Go to the nearest house with lights on and pound on the door for help. Don't worry about appearing silly if it turns out to be a false alarm. Even if your fears are unwarranted, feeling silly is a small price to pay for keeping yourself safe.

If you must walk alone at night—to get back and forth to a job, for instance—assume a confident attitude and a determined walking stance that says you know exactly where you're going and plan to get there quickly. Then do so. If night walking is a necessity or if you just want to feel as confident as possible throughout the day, you may want to take a self-defense course, and Debby highly recommends a program called Model Mugging. (See Appendix for more details.) And if you do have the misfortune to be attacked, report it to the police if you feel able to because that could alert them to the presence of someone who might attack other women too. If you don't want to talk to the police, you can still seek help from a local rape crisis or women's center or from one of the victims-of-crime programs emerging in larger urban areas. Do not *ever* assume that you were at fault or that you should be able to deal with the psychological trauma of an attack by yourself. You need never deal with such an experience alone. There is help available.

Running May Be Just Your Thing

So many millions of words have been written about running during the last ten years that you'd think we'd invented it rather than inheriting it from our ancestors in the caves. Writers wax poetic about its benefits to mind, body, and spirit and, to be sure, it can be a wonderfully empowering, exhilarating experience. Skimming across the earth is an almost primal kind of excitement, and slow, long-distance running can be mesmerizing. For some of us, part of the enticement of running is that it is thought to be dangerous or even impossible for fat people. Those of us who scoff at rules made for mere mortals may be mobilized by this factor alone. While running is not for everyone and is actually diminishing in popularity in part because of injury rates, every year nearly one hundred thousand people are still attracted to the Bay to Breakers race in San Francisco, and millions of women wouldn't trade their running shoes for anything. So it could be just the challenge you are looking for. You may actually run slower than you walk, but running feels different from walking and captures the spirit of sport in a way that may entice you.

If you decide to take up running, it's best to buy a book specifically about it for advice and guidance because even though our cave parents did it, our modern bodies have forgotten how. One of the best books is Dr. Joan Ullyot's first book, *Women's Running* (see Appendix). Although she is wedded to the idea of practically fat-free bodies, Ullyot does cover the most important issues beginning women runners need to know, and you can read around her fat phobia. If you start running before you buy a book for help, the walking tips given earlier are also applicable to running. Be sure to include adequate time to warm up, cool down, and stretch in your routine. Large women should also pay particular attention to monitoring their heart rate and buying shoes and bras designed specifically for running. (Refer to Chapter 3 for advice on buying shoes.)

If you start running after being in a walking program for a while, the transition to running can be gradual. You can begin by alternating walking with running—walk five minutes, run two, walk ten minutes, run five, back and forth until your running and walking times are about equal and then gradually increase your running time and decrease your walking time, allowing your body to get used to the change. This way you build up strength over time and lessen your risk of injury. You will progress more quickly if you set a time goal, say, 30 to 45 minutes, and walk/run for the entire time, rather than just running as far as you can and then quitting.

Remember to stay within your target heart rate whether walking or running. You will need to monitor this by taking your pulse or the "talk test" described in the Walking Tips section. While you can safely skip monitoring your heart rate if your walks are leisurely, it is not at all wise to skip it when running. There is absolutely no point in overchallenging your heart and getting into trouble. Any chest pain is a signal to *stop* immediately, rest, and then get medical attention. Shortness of breath, dizziness, nausea, and light-headedness are also signs of overexertion and should be respected as signals to slow down to stop.

Running is not encouraged for larger people because of the concern for potential cardiovascular risk and because of the impact greater weight places on your feet and joints. When you run, the impact on your feet and joints is that of approximately three times your body weight. If you weigh two hundred pounds, this is six hundred pounds of pressure on each foot with each step. While this may not be a problem at first, over time it could create difficulty. But you must be the judge about what you want to try, and you may be able to run safely if you are informed about the risks and take adequate precautions. It is especially important to have shoes with excellent support and cushioning to absorb the shock, and these shoes will tend to be in the upper price range. They're worth it. Once you find the right shoes, it is also best to run on a surface that "gives" rather than on concrete or blacktop even if this means running around a dirt track at a local school.

You will want to become especially adept at tuning into your body's messages so you can tell if particular muscles or joints are getting ready to cause you problems. It will be important for you to learn the difference between a dull aching-type pain, which may be from simply overdoing it, and the sharp pain that is a possible sign of injury. While there are times when humans can "run through pain and go to a higher level," why risk it? Pain is a message from the body, and we should listen to it so that exercise is pleasure, not punishment. "No pain, no gain" may be the worst advice ever given to exercisers. Slow down or stop when your body sends the pain message. Any persistent pain should be checked out by a sports medicine professional for suggestions on altering stride, correcting any shoe problems you have, doing exercises to strengthen specific muscle groups, or dealing with any other issues pertinent to your needs.

I Wanna Take You Higher

There are few experiences more exhilarating than working your way through trees and shrubs, around rocks and boulders, and turning a corner or coming to the top of a hill and looking out over an incredible vista. Purple mountains' majesty is not just a line in a song. Hiking is a sport growing in popularity not only because it is physically challenging and invigorating but because it can land you in the middle of the wilderness, Mother Nature's gift to us all. Whether you hike in a city park and have to block out the traffic sounds to let your imagination soar to the mountain tops or you actually make it to the mountaintops, hiking is a direct way of connecting with the earth. Even a couple of hours out among the trees and birds can soothe any nagging stresses and help put troubling issues into perspective. It is also great fun. Take a lunch and your favorite book, and a whole day can whiz by. If you're lucky you can snag a kid to go with you and turn you on to the wonders you might just miss on your own.

If you're hiking in a wilderness area, it's best to go with a friend, particularly if you are a beginner. A cruise around a local park with well-marked, highly traveled trails is one thing, but if you are going into unfamiliar territory where trail traffic is light, carry a map (that you've learned how to read) and tell another friend or someone at a ranger station of your expected route and approximate time of return. After working as a nurse in Yosemite National Park, I think I've seen almost every injury possible in the mountains, some serious enough to cause death, and many if not most of them could have been prevented. It's amazing how frequently people used to flat, urban areas jump out of their cars in the mountains and naively and unnecessarily run into trouble. It is no embarrassment not to know the ropes in the mountains, and it's important to keep in mind that the only stupid question is the one that's not asked. There are informed people and trail guidebooks at most visitor's centers, paid for by your tax dollars, by the way. Get the most out of them.

Go slower than usual until you get acclimated to any increase in altitude and check your pulse rate more frequently to be sure you're not overdoing it. Increased altitude creates increased physical stress because there is less oxygen available. The "talk test" can still be your guide. The potential for freak storms in mountain areas means you should always check the weather report before you depart and carry a pack with water, some food such as cheese, nuts, and fruit, and a heavier sweater or jacket. Sunscreen, insect repellent, and moleskin (to prevent blisters) are also good to have along. Stay on marked trails and consider any animal you encounter to be wild. Deer are not friendly little Bambis just waiting for you to pet them, and bears take very unkindly to humans messing with their cubs no matter how cute and curious they are. Common sense can be a good basic guide to enjoying yourself, but do check out books about hiking or backpacking for more complete and specific information. Experienced companions are the best insurance for safety and a good time.

Whether walking, running, or hiking, you will get some exercise, some fresh air, and a challenge if you wish. You may even find inspiration. The confidence that comes from knowing you can walk or run a good distance is subtle but powerful. Once while driving with a friend on a back road that was far from our destination (lost, in other words), I realized that even if we ran out of gas I'd be okay. I'd survive because I could walk out if I absolutely had to. While that never became necessary, I realized what an effective antidote to panic I had developed. I now have the confidence to go camping in remote areas, ones that I otherwise might have avoided. I can also run to catch a bus when I need to without fearing I'll have a heart attack right there on the street. Simply being able to walk can give you more confidence and make much more accessible parts of the world you never thought you'd see.

Let's Make Waves

A few years ago several women in the Bay Area had a simple but brilliant idea: rent time at a local pool and set up a swim session for large women only. Voila! A safe place was created where all sizes of larger women would feel totally welcome, comfortable, and free to be themselves. Now, a day at the Saturday swim is a regular and

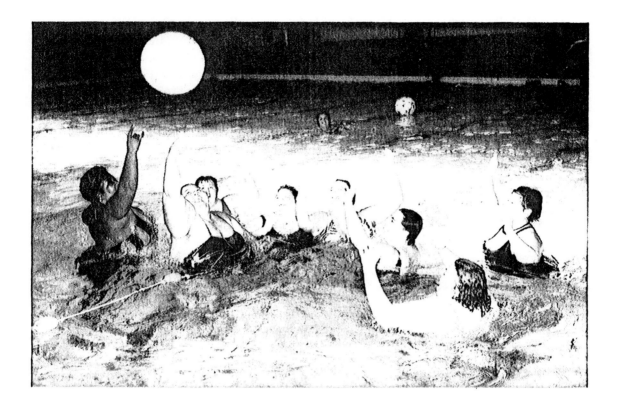

incredibly empowering part of many women's lives. Fat women have been told forever that we look so ugly in swimsuits (if we could even find one to fit) that we should spare the world the distress of seeing us. Some of us have spent summers indoors or under blankets to avoid the painfully cold reception we get at virtually every swimming occasion. No more, we say!

At the swim we are free to enjoy the sensuous pleasure of the water without worrying about putdowns. One regular swimmer said she would never have had the confidence to go to Hawaii, hang out on the beach, and swim to her heart's content had she not become comfortable and more self-accepting of her body in a bathing suit after two years at the swim. Special swim groups like this have been established in other parts of the country, and you and your friends might consider organizing one in your area. All it takes is several interested women committed to the idea and willing to do some work to make it happen. It will be well worth the effort.

The optimum pool is one with warm water and stairs, not just ladders, for getting in and out. Stairs enable women whose mobility is limited, either by their size or by a physically limiting condition such as arthritis, to participate more easily. Once you have chosen a pool, arrange for a specific amount of time when your group can pay for a lifeguard to be available. (The Saturday Swim charges each swimmer $2 to $5, depending on ability to pay, and uses this money to pay for pool rental.) If pool managers are skeptical about whether you can get enough women to warrant the time, assure them you plan a publicity effort. If it is a public pool (as most are), remind the manager that your swimmers are taxpayers too. Once arrangements for the pool are made, design an eye-catching flyer and distribute it everywhere you can think of—large women's clothing stores, women's centers, and book stores. Give flyers to all of your friends to pass on to large women they know. It takes some patience and ongoing determination, but you will love the results.

During the two-hour Saturday swim in the Bay Area, women swim laps, play volleyball, stretch, and walk around in the pool, using the water for resistance, or simply hang out and enjoy each other's company. It can be a time to share information on goods and services for larger women or just catch up on the latest happenings in people's lives. It can be a great place to let people know you're looking for work or child care, or just laugh yourself silly and play around. One regular says that while she doesn't swim laps or play games for specific exercise, simply being in the water encourages her to move and stretch, and she has become more relaxed and flexible as a result. Most important, it feels marvelous to come together to swim vigorously or just have fun without having to brace yourself for the put-downs so often associated with swimming. Some women who have learned to love swimming in this safe environment now venture into other pools and experiences with much more confidence, as our Hawaii vacationer can attest. But remember, regardless of where you swim, you have the right to be in any pool or on any beach you choose and be treated with respect.

One difficult aspect of creating these large-women-only environments is arriving at a definition of "large." With virtually every woman in America thinking she is too fat even when she actually may be anorexically thin, self-definition alone seems inadequate. For instance, a woman who is ten pounds "overweight" according to insurance company tables may think she is fat even if she is not, and she certainly does not face the level of public prejudice and discrimination that a woman who weighs three hundred pounds does. Smaller women can and do make life considerably worse for larger women by using them as a way to feel better about themselves, saying: "Thank god I'm not that fat." In fact, they are part of the problem that creates the need for fat-women-only swims in the first place! But where exactly is the cutoff point? If two hundred pounds is used, some shorter women who are fat but will never weigh that much are excluded. Since fat women constantly have suffered prejudice and exclusion, there is reluctance to contribute to the problem by perpetuating any unnecessary "us and them" divisions.

In discussing this issue in one of their newsletters, Ample Opportunity, a health organization for fat women in Portland, Oregon, has struggled with this issue while designing a variety of activity programs for women—belly dance classes, swims, cross-country ski trips, camping, and so forth. "We have found this issue to be highly charged. . . . It is very difficult to deal with in a way that protects the *balance* of rights and sensitivities of a range of fat women. . . . We want to define our center and not deny our edges. We want to enlist the most people possible in assuring a good quality of life irrespective of body type. . . . We have not found a way to do this which does not hurt some fat women or make others anxious and unwilling to participate." As the concern to create safe exercise space for larger women grows, this is an issue that groups will continually have to wrestle with.

Can $6.95 Change Your Life?

Personally, I used to loathe the idea of lap swimming for exercise—ugh, how boring. I grew up taking free, city-sponsored swim lessons and became a relatively competent swimmer at a young age. I was even one of twenty young bathing beauties who performed oh-so-graceful synchronized swim routines, à la Esther Williams movies, for the end-of-summer gala swim show. Parents were kind enough to attend and applaud grandly. Once I got a little older it became much more important to me and my girl friends to lounge around on the grass next to the pool, working on a tan to *look* sexy and healthy rather than mess our hair and *be* healthy from swimming. I felt much more self-conscious than sexy in these situations but became adept at hiding any hurt or uncomfortable feelings. I did begin to think of swimming and water ballet antics as kid's stuff, though, and besides, I hated getting all that chlorine in my eyes and up my nose. No fun and definitely uncool. Aside from some water skiing and a little splashing around occasionally in lakes in my twenties and thirties, I was a has-been swimmer, and it didn't bother me a bit.

Even after I started going to the Saturday swim I still had a lot of resistance to swimming laps. I always swam with my head out of the water to avoid all the spitting and coughing that seemed inevitable with swimming most lap strokes, but I developed a terrible crick in my neck and ended up spitting up water anyway. Then a simple little $6.95 purchase of swim goggles made it a whole new ball game. All of a sudden I was twelve again, full of adventure, able to swim underwater and not crash into other swimmers. I actually began to like having my face in the water because I could see, and I began to imagine how much fun scuba diving must be. Being able to see all the other bodies moving underwater added to the appeal, and I could steal swim tips from the other swimmers whenever I wanted by just watching them and trying to do what they were doing. Finally, I decided I wanted to learn the breathing necessary to swim laps with my face in the water.

Learning the regular, relaxed breathing that's part of the crawl, the most common lap swimming stroke, takes a few lessons and a lot of practice, but once you get the hang of it, it is a great form of meditation that you can do almost indefinitely. In essence it is the same kind of very shallow breathing in your upper lungs that you do when you are sleeping. Instead of trying to take deep full breaths, which will wear you out in short order, swimming the crawl involves taking very shallow gulps of air out of one side of your mouth while you keep the other side of your face resting against the water. Then you blow the air out underwater while continuing to stroke. It is this regular breathe-stroke-breathe-stroke rhythm that can put you into a virtual trance if you do it long enough.

Because this breathing is tricky to master, try practicing before you actually begin to swim laps. Stand in shallow water or float with your face in the water while grasping the side of the pool. Concentrate on slow, regular breathing to establish a rhythm and try to be aware of exactly how the breathing motion feels. For instance, does your face feel as if it is gently resting against the water? Is your neck relaxed, allowing your head to turn easily to the side for air and then into the water? Is your mouth just barely out of the water when you take your small breath? Are you able to blow the air out through your nose and mouth at the same time? Once you get a rhythm down and are tuned into exactly how you feel during practice, it is easier to begin swimming, concentrating most on the feeling of your breathing motion while practicing and trying to reproduce that feeling. When you begin swimming, go as slowly as you possibly can while you master this breathing technique. If you have problems with learning this breathing, ask an instructor or lifeguard at your swim to watch you and give you tips on what to work on. You might even wish to invest in a few lessons. Eventually, you may find, as I did, that, with practice, swimming becomes a whole new adventure.

Now I can cruise along with a backstroke (it feels great to open up my chest and stretch my shoulders and upper back), switch to a few laps of the crawl (fun to try in very slow, medium, and fast gears), glide through the water with a sidestroke, do underwater exploring with the breaststroke, on and on until I have stretched and moved my body every way possible. Swimming laps using different strokes has become a way to get aerobic exercise while moving all of my body in a balanced way not possible in other activities. I'm not just using my right side as in tennis or softball, for instance, or my legs as in walking. Using different kicking and arm stroking styles, practically every muscle in my body can get stronger and more flexible. After a few laps doing a sidestroke on my right side, for instance, I can switch to my left and try to become equally adept. It felt clumsy at first, but the more I do it the more natural it feels and the more I learn about moving on both sides in a more evenly balanced way.

Like most pools, mine has a clock, so rather than aiming for a set number of laps I have a time goal. I started with 30 seconds nonstop, now go for about 20 minutes, and am aiming for more. Another swimmer starts out with lots of rubber bands on one wrist, each representing one lap. As she swims she transfers a rubber band from one wrist to the other until all the rubber bands end up on her other wrist. And certainly some swimmers say the hell with counting laps or minutes and just go at it for as long as it feels right. This is truly a case of different strokes for different folks.

As with any aerobic activity, if you keep at it your strength and endurance will build and you can only surpass your former goals. One Saturday swimmer over fifty years of age, immobilized by arthritis just a few years ago, now swims 40 minutes nonstop three times a week and says she is a new person. It has literally changed her life, freeing her from both immobility and pain. She is an inspiration for the rest of us.

As far as swimming being an ideal exercise for larger women, it is true that body fat aids rather than hinders the process. Fat floats, so just lying there in suspended animation is incredibly relaxing in itself. It's wonderful to escape gravity. If you decide to move, the water does not put any stress on your joints but does create a helpful kind of resistance to build muscle strength. Swimming gives many people a way to feel sensuous and graceful right from the start, without ever having to worry about falling down and breaking a leg.

For people who have not yet learned to swim or who are a bit rusty, proper instruction is immensely helpful, and classes are usually offered at YM or YWCAs. In addition there are often classes that combine stretching and strengthening exercises with a variety of movements to do at an aerobic pace in the water. Once you learn the routines you can do them yourself or simply continue going to the classes. As usual, going with a friend, particularly another fat woman, makes it psychologically easier at first and more fun. However, you don't have to swim laps to get aerobic exercise; you can simply walk in the water at a speed that will get your heart rate up to your target rate for as long as you decide to keep going. But don't let any limiting attitudes stop you from swimming laps if you want to try. Most pools that offer lap swimming either give you your own lane or divide the pool into slow, medium, and fast lanes shared by swimmers who go at the same pace. And don't be worried about being too slow for even the slow lane. Your fellow swimmers will simply pass you, just as faster drivers do on the freeway. There's no need to feel embarrassed about your pace, whatever it is.

For maximum overall benefit, model your swimming routine on the one described earlier for walking: warm-up, exercise, cool-down, stretch. Pay particular attention to stretches for your arms and upper body since swimming is one of the only forms of exercise that really stresses and thus strengthens these muscles. You may want to buy a book about swimming, which will no doubt include a full stretching program for this sport.

If you are bothered by tension in your shoulders and upper back during your exercise routine, try floating on your back with your arms pointed straight over your head and then kick your way across the pool. Alternate this move with your other strokes. Be particularly aware of any movements that place stress on your lower back, such as using float boards to practice your kicking. While this works fine for some as a way to isolate and practice kicking movements, others find it places too much strain on the lower back. The more you become aware of how your body feels in motion, the more you will be able to tailor your routine to what feels best.

One barrier to swimming has always been finding a bathing suit in a large enough size, one that was made for actually swimming and not just for sitting on the sidelines. Fortunately, Big Stitches by Jan is a business created to respond to this overwhelming need. Jan makes suits in fabulous colors and styles, in sizes 38 to 60. She has in one fell swoop freed fat women swimmers to express themselves with color and design not possible until she came along. (Jan's address is listed in the Appendix so that you, too, can get one of these marvelous suits.) Maybe department stores and other swimsuit designers will catch on to the idea soon. Once you have your suit you're ready to go with just a few more words before you plunge ahead:

Try swim goggles. When you first go to a store to buy goggles it's hard to know which kind are going to be comfortable without trying them on. Some stores will let you do this while others will not. And some people are wary of trying them on without using some sort of disinfectant such as alcohol (which stores may also resist your using before purchase). You may simply have to try the most popular brand recommended by the sales clerk, unless of course they're pushing the $25 kind. There's no need to spend that much since perfectly adequate goggles cost less than $10, and when you forget them at the pool sometime, which inevitably happens, you won't be out a big investment.

If you and the store are comfortable with trying goggles on before purchase, hold them up to your eyes with a little pressure and then see if they stay in place without your having to use the strap. If they fall off, try another type. The rubber strap is not meant to be the only thing anchoring goggles to your head. Both the rubber strap and the nose piece can be adjusted to fit you comfortably once you get eyepieces that fit. The eyepieces should be surrounded by enough foam padding for comfort and so that you won't get a headache, and they should have anti-fog lenses. To further ensure visibility, rub the insides of your lenses with saliva before going in the water, then rinse them out with pool water. Or buy one of the special defogging solutions available in sporting goods shops and at many pools.

Swimming is a lot more fun if you can see while you do it. If you're able to see the lane dividers painted on the bottom of the pool, you'll also be able to stay in a straight line while swimming and avoid a concussion from ramming into other swimmers.

Taking a quick pulse can substitute for the talk test. Because you can't take the talk test while you're swimming, if you are interested in getting maximal aerobic benefits you will want to take your pulse periodically to be sure you are swimming within your aerobic target rate.* Learn to take a quick pulse for six seconds and multiply by ten.

Drink enough water.   Be sure you drink enough before and after your swim to keep yourself well hydrated. Even though you may be in water that feels cool, your body will still heat up and sweat the longer you swim, so you need to replace the lost fluid. Many people get extremely thirsty while swimming. The warmer the water and the greater the amount of chlorination, the more water you will need to drink. Keep an extra jug of water in your car to sip on your way to and from your swim.

If you think swimming laps in a pool can get boring, you can try open water swimming, which is what Lynne Cox decided to do. Saying she just got tired swimming laps back and forth and wanted to *get* somewhere, at age fifteen Cox broke and rebroke the men's and women's world records for swimming the twenty-one-mile English Channel. She kept swimming and kept looking for challenges. On August 7, 1987, at the ripe old age of thirty, Cox completed the coldest swim in history. With only her swimsuit and cap between her body and the near freezing 40-degree water, she swam the 2.7-mile Bering Strait between Alaska and the USSR in just over two hours. (Because of the currents, she actually ended up swimming over four miles.) She was welcomed by Russians in full picnic mode to celebrate her record-setting, teeth-chattering crossing.

What is the reason I mention Cox here? Right. Her body has been called perfect for the sport of distance swimming because she is five feet six inches tall, weighs 209 pounds, and has a body fat percentage of 40, nearly twice the 22 percent women are told to aim for "ideally." Cox's accomplishments are awe-inspiring, period. But she also shatters stereotypes about large women's potential for health and peak conditioning, doesn't she. We'll no doubt hear more about her in the coming years as she continues to *get* somewhere. Three cheers, Lynne. Way to go!

When I watched the 1984 Olympics I found that my old love, synchronized swimming, was being revived and turned into an Olympic event. The strength and coordination it takes were obvious (to say nothing of the swimmers' ability to hold their breath forever

---

*Recent research indicates that because our bodies stay cool in water even when they are working aerobically, our hearts beat about 15 beats/minute slower. Therefore the target heart rate for swimming is 205 minus your age, multiplied by .7, and for a six-second count, divided by 10. For a 40-year old: 205 − 40 = 165. 165 × .7 = 116. 116 div. by 10 = 12.

while doing amazing underwater maneuvers), and I remembered how easily I'd rejected it years before as kid's stuff. I'm delighted to have rediscovered swimming after all these years because it is so invigorating and cleansing at the same time. While I may never jump into icy water, all my dolphin fantasies can take me on grand trips in my mind, while slow, rhythmic breathing puts my mind in perfectly relaxed unison with my body.

Playing volleyball in the water is a vigorous way to top off the morning, particularly if the game is geared to keeping the ball in motion as long as possible. While on land I seem bolted to the ground and unable to jump higher than a fraction of an inch, in the water I shed my earth-bound gravity-induced limitations. I can leap and soar and reach even the hardest to hit shots because I know when I fall it will be a soft landing. And when I look around the Saturday swim and see all the other big, strong, beautiful women in a rainbow of swimsuit colors and styles, well, I just feel happy. And being happy is a big part of being healthy.

If you've never thought of walking, running, or swimming as activities you could do, perhaps these pages have encouraged you to try one or the other of them. If you never thought of these activities as sports or of yourself as a sporting type, then you may have had too limited a vision of both. Give yourself a chance. You may start out walking on level ground but, who knows, you may end up in high mountain places. That's what happened to me—and believe me, I was as surprised as anyone when I found myself there!

Mountain Magic

I once thought only a crazy person would put forty pounds of equipment on her back and voluntarily walk up a hill, let alone trek into the mountains. Whizzing down ski slopes in the mountains was one thing; there was a chair lift to do the hard work of getting back up the mountain. Even when I lived in the glory of Yosemite National Park for a year during my early twenties and any walk could have been visually rewarding, I always drove the two blocks to the grocery store rather than walk, and I thought hiking was something only nature nuts could appreciate. Besides, the stereotype of fat women as not strong or fit enough for the sport of backpacking had been with me for a long time. With the help of my friend Jeanne, a sturdy mountain woman with a taste for Yukon Jack and a ten-year love affair with fresh air at high altitudes, I got a chance to change my mind on all counts.

As a thirty-sixth birthday present to myself, Jeanne, her friend Mike, and I planned a four-day trip into the Sierra Nevada mountains of California, a trip that included two mountain passes over ten thousand feet. Since I loved camping and had been running for three years, Jeanne said that not only was I in good enough shape to do it with no sweat but I'd love it. I believed her.

With borrowed hiking boots and backpack, neither of which fit me particularly well, we began our trip. We had to cross the first pass at about three miles. No dillydallying around getting acclimated! Just hop right to it. People do this for fun? I had never carried so much weight on my back and began questioning the need for food, clothing, sleeping bag, and other presumed necessities. If littering the trail with my belongings had been at all acceptable, I would have dumped them on the spot. The seven miles we covered that day blistered my feet and battered my enthusiasm and confidence.

The second day was worse. By four o'clock, after Jeanne had said at least three times that the campsite she had in mind was "just a little farther," I had a serious case of *attitude*—anger, irritability, and despair. Could the rangers please send in the helicopter to get me? Why did I ever consent to this? Worst of all was the feeling of being a drag to Jeanne and Mike who, hard as it was for me to believe, truly seemed to be enjoying themselves immensely. Although I managed to keep my verbal complaints to a minimum, I wasn't kidding anyone. My shlumping downhill shuffle was matched by my less-than-chamber-of-commerce-bright smile.

By the time we reached our long-awaited campsite, even with my bad attitude, I had to admit it was indeed perfect. Of course I would have gladly camped in a grocery store parking lot at that point, so the rushing stream with a waterfall, surrounded by wild flowers of every color in the rainbow, was just what a travel bureau might have promised—sheer mountain magic.

Certainly it must be true that the quiet splendor of the mountains is healing, a soothing rejuvenation for the soul (if not the soles). On the third day my pack seemed much lighter and my blisters much less bothersome, and I found myself beginning to really enjoy the body strain and the challenge. Me, enjoying going uphill, stressing my body? As we approached the steepest part of our journey I was stoked and ready. I remembered skills I'd studied in sport psychology that had worked to master other difficult physical challenges and knew that if I could just shift my attention to an internal focus on my body, it would be a lot easier.

As the trail got steeper with each step, I concentrated more and more on my breathing, visualizing myself as a strong mountain creature able to blend with the switchbacks and curves leading to the top. The rocks, trees, flowers, birds, and streams became a chorus of encouragement. The sound that seemed the loudest, though, was my breathing, slow and rhythmic. My legs felt so strong and my breathing so easy that I felt I could have walked forever. When the trail began to level off I was a bit in awe of the strong body I had never before realized was mine, and I had a pang of regret that there was no more uphill left in my sweaty dance with Mother Nature. I was babbling happily when Jeanne and Mike caught up with me. "No wonder you love this," I said.

Afterwards I realized that concentrating on my breathing and visualizing my legs and lungs as members of a team working in unison had worked as a meditation to keep my focus in the present, away from such distracting and demoralizing thoughts as, "How much farther?" I found that even if my body seemed to falter, a positive attitude and a focus of concentration on specific aspects of my movement came to my rescue when it really counted. Concentrating on, rather than ignoring my body enabled me to enjoy and accomplish a real challenge. What's more, I now know where I can find this extra dose of help whenever I need it to learn any other new sport—it's as close as my next breath. And to think I could have missed it all by not trying!

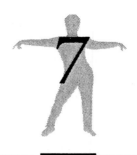

Sports for Any Body (Yes, This Means You!)

Does the memory of PE give you heartburn or bring tears to your eyes even today? So many adults seem able to relate painful or embarrassing childhood experiences of PE with such vivid instant recall—of teachers or the other kids ridiculing them for being too fat or too slow, or of being picked last, if at all, for teams—that one wonders sometimes who was enjoying the playing. If you carry any emotional scars from such experiences, it is no surprise if you are wary when someone says, "Hey, come on, you can do it!" Ironically, even if you were athletic while growing up, you may still have had to put up with ridicule because athletic girls were often called tomboys and not thought of as "real girls." Fortunately, as adults we can act from the knowledge of who we are today and not remain stalled in youthful memories, however uncomfortable they may be.

If you think sports are just for lean people with highly developed muscles and a super competitive attitude, we want you to reconsider. We'd like to help you overcome any attitude or past experience that limits the vision of your possibilities. No matter how much you weigh or how many years it's been since you've played, you do not have to settle for inactivity. Large women swim, run, hike, cycle, canoe, camp, ski, do martial arts, and play tennis, softball, volleyball, and practically any other sport you can name. You can, too, if you wish. You may just have to overcome some of what you learned in PE to do so.

We Dance enthusiast Cheryl White's experience is not atypical: "A few years ago I read a book called *The Ultimate Athlete* [by George Leonard] and was surprised to find out that most people have had a PE experience which was very uncomfortable. With so much competition they grew to hate movement and never wanted to move again after they got out of school. I was surprised because that's just what happened to me in school. I never remember being taught how to throw a ball or how to do things, I was just tested. And I always failed because I was never *taught,* never coached. I always had pretty good coordination, but because of my family life I thought I was huge and a freak; in reality I was just a few pounds overweight for a kid. When I look back, one of the things that would have brought my sense of my body back into proportion was a really good education in physical movement. And I never got that."

Even if you never had the chance when growing up to have a good education in physical movement, you can begin now. People love sports, not just for the fun to be had but because often, unexpectedly, a sport experience can bowl you over with inspiration. Physical activity done with attention to body awareness can also be a healing force to improve your sense of confidence in your body and thus improve your body image. In these pages you'll see how some of the limited attitudes toward women in sport have affected us all. You'll learn about developing a more playful attitude and hear from larger women with a variety of reasons for getting started in a particular sport. Most of all, we hope you'll learn that if you want to play, you can.

The Thrill of Victory and the Agony of PE—A Brief History of Women in Sport

When Joan Benoit crossed the finish line of the 1984 Olympic marathon and ran her victory lap, grinning and crying, women all over the world cried with her, cheered and danced in celebration. It was a little hard to breathe with so much pride swelling our chests. Benoit won the race and in the process scored a victory for all women. She and the hundreds of thousands of women athletes all over the world were living proof that women's potential for achievement in sport is limited only by the barriers created by sexism.

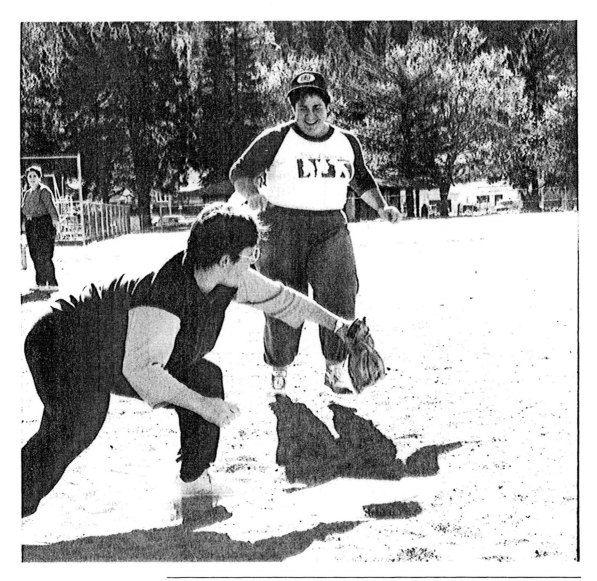

Oakland Raters Cheron Dudley and Alice Ansfield take time out from walking to try a little softball.

Since the days of the original Olympic games in Greece, women have been told that we have neither the strength nor the endurance to run the 26.2-mile marathon distance. Women were banned "for our own protection" from running in this Olympic event. (Women are still banned by the Olympic Committee from running the ten thousand meters.) We were also told that to be a skilled athlete was inherently unfeminine. Fear of being labeled lesbian has probably kept millions of women, regardless of their sexuality, from any involvement in sports. Fortunately, sport-loving women, both lesbian and straight, have persisted in spite of the discrimination such fear can create and in spite of the divisiveness it can perpetuate among women. They have worked to change attitudes toward women participants and to improve opportunities for all sporting women and girls. Given the task, their efforts have been incredibly successful. In order to appreciate what women are still up against, the battle to celebrate physical competence and strength as positive qualities of healthy women is one that must be viewed in its historical context.

The idea of women as emotionally frail and physically ill equipped for strenuous exercise and competition has existed at least since 776 B.C. when the women of Greece were not allowed to watch, much less participate, in Olympic events. Physical prowess did not fit with popular definitions of femininity among the Greeks. In the days of the Roman Empire, women still were not allowed to play but were allowed to watch and cheer male participants. In effect they became the forerunners of the Dallas Cowboys' cheerleaders.

In a historical fast-forward move, we can examine the Victorian era of the nineteenth century, where the upper class woman was assumed to be naturally weak and passive and her "place" restricted to the pedestal. While an occasional game of bowling or croquet was considered acceptable for women of the leisure class, participation in anything more active was controlled so that they would not appear unladylike. (Sweat? Madam, please, restrain thyself!) During this same time period, women of lower socioeconomic classes were too busy working to find themselves on pedestals or sporting fields. (This class difference still exists today. Middle and upper class white women are the predominant participants in collegiate athletics and private fitness clubs, while workingclass women and women of color are overrepresented in the ranks of those who have neither enough time nor disposable income to participate fully in fitness and sport activities.)

In 1917, according to women's sports writer Stephanie Twin, "the most widely approved form of female physical activity was physical culture: mild calisthenics designed to strengthen, beautify, or correct various parts of the body. . . . Her body, a means to social ends—beauty, motherhood, education—rather than something to be mastered in itself, simply needed to be kept healthy. . . . Few suggested that through sports women might gain mastery over their bodies, and most doubted even that they could." During World War

I, women mastered many of the physically demanding jobs that were necessarily vacated by men. Thus, after the war, their confidence bolstered by their obvious physical abilities and potential, women became much more involved in competitive athletics. Swimming, tennis, ice skating, and golf became popular in the twenties and thirties, and by 1936 basketball was the most popular women's sport.

But it was also in the late 1920s and early 1930s that physical educators began to protest that competition was exploitation. Twin reports "educators claimed that women were being pushed beyond themselves, physically and emotionally, to satisfy crowds . . . predicting that nervous instability, premature pelvic ossification, narrowed vaginas, difficult deliveries, heart strain, and spinsterhood were the high prices women would pay for being serious contenders." (You laugh. They believed this! Some people today may still believe it.)

Under the guise of "protection," women's participation in society has always been historically curtailed. So it's not surprising that competitive sports were purposefully eliminated from women's physical education "for our own good." The rigidity of sex roles was maintained on the sporting fields as well as in the rest of society— men are strong; women need strong protectors rather than to become strong ourselves. The result was a sharp decline in the numbers of women involved in sport between the 1930s and 1970s. While there have always been accomplished female athletes willing to challenge the status quo, athletic opportunities for the vast majority of women were squelched by the determined neglect and even hostility of educational institutions. Calisthenics "to tone and beautify the body" became the essence of most women's physical education. Sports became almost exclusively male territory.

Competitive sports are traditionally viewed as a way to strengthen both muscle and moral fiber, and have been hailed by the likes of General MacArthur as a true testing ground for the character development necessary for soldiers in battle. (It's obvious he was not thinking about female character!) American sports have a distinctly military flavor—with the national anthem at the start of every contest, marching bands, an opposing team called "the enemy," and the "kill 'em" chant before the game. The sports establishment emphasizes individual achievement, competitiveness, a Protestant work-ethic brand of discipline and, most of all, winning. It is precisely these values that are the foundation of capitalist society and commercial success. Therefore, to change any of the attitudes and values of the sporting world is tantamount to changing society. As it happens, that is precisely what women set out to do in their renewed search for equality during the 1970s. That is one reason for women's increased participation in sports since then.

One event in 1973 stands out vividly in my mind as a touchstone of changing social perceptions about women's abilities in sport: the trouncing tennis defeat Billie Jean King served to Bobby Riggs. An aging tennis star always looking for a way to make a buck promoting himself, Riggs claimed he could beat even the top women tennis players of the day and that women's tennis was too boring to be given much respect, let alone much prize money. He beat Wimbledon champ Margaret Court and boasted unmercifully. Then Billie Jean took up his challenge.

Throughout the land, men and women waged bets on who would win, lining up in almost strict gender ranks. When the much ballyhooed match took place on national television, King beat the socks off Riggs in three straight sets. Perhaps no other victory in her enormously successful career, encompassing twenty Wimbledon championships, established King's status as an inspiring hero to women, even those uninterested in sport, as much as this one. She accepted a challenge from a man on his turf and won. Many men's worst fears about women's participation in sport were realized—yes, on a given day a woman could beat a man at his own game, and the world would go on turning. What a concept.

King and other women athletes went on to found the Virginia Slims women's tennis tour (increasing both the purse and respect for women's tennis in the process), the Women's Sports Foundation, and *Women's Sports* magazine, blazing a trail for other women and girls to follow. But King's victory over Riggs remains an especially amusing memory, particularly given the fact that some men were absolutely convinced that Riggs had thrown the match! Undaunted, and with determined smiles, women declared we were in the world of sport to stay.

In 1972, legal battles finally won passage of Title IX federal legislation and forced institutions to give women equal access (but certainly not equal funding) to sports. Passage of this legislation coincided with the fitness boom of the mid 1970s to produce a dramatic rise in the number of women participants in all physical activities. In 1972 there were 101,859 girls and women playing softball on teams registered with the Amateur Softball Association; in 1983, 5.4 million of us played organized softball. Ten years ago there were fewer than 1 million female runners in the U.S.; today there are over 19 million. Ten years ago no statistics even existed on participation in aerobics; today 15 million people participate, 95 percent of whom are women. The number of women participating in the Olympics rose from 781 in 1968 to 1,681 in 1984. Sweating, the bane of our Victorian grandmothers, is now fashionable!

Anyone who has watched Martina Navratilova serve a tennis ball or Cheryl Miller slam dunk a basketball or ice skater Debi Thomas nail a perfect triple loop knows that women who dedicate themselves to their sport can be thrilling to watch. They can inspire little girls and adult women everywhere to do their best at whatever they try. Competitive sports need not drain a woman of her desire for fun nor deprive her of any sense of her femininity. But women still must put up with being told they "play tennis like a man" as if that were the highest compliment, and there are still women not totally comfortable beating a man at any game, even if it's only a Sunday afternoon tennis outing. Battles continue to rage about whether boys and girls should be allowed to compete against each other or play on the same teams. Until winning is put into its proper perspective—and not viewed as a necessary outcome in order for men to retain self-esteem when competing with women or viewed as a way for women to derive an exaggerated sense of self-esteem in encounters with men—these battles will persist. Women don't get involved in sports in order to beat men, but we do want the opportunity to play and to become stronger and better at whatever game we choose.

But rules of conduct about what is considered masculine and feminine stubbornly persist, which may explain why more women in the 1980s suit up in matching leotards and tights than in a softball jersey. Sports that emphasize speed, strength, power, and teamwork are still felt to be unfamiliar territory to many women, despite all the years, dollars, and words spent in court fights and the blood, sweat, and tears women athletes, coaches, and educators have shed to open the playing fields to all of us. Somehow, to be a woman and competent at sports, particularly competitive sports, is still considered suspect on the femininity scale. Equally as disappointing is the fact that sport participation is still considered the domain of only the serious athlete. No apologies should be necessary for the woman who wants to be a serious contender or for the woman who wants to be a fun-and-games recreational athlete.

To make matters worse, the goal of weight loss remains an underlying motivating factor for many, regardless of what activity is chosen, harkening back to 1917 when we women were supposed to concentrate on beautifying ourselves and correcting our bodily flaws. Fat is definitely viewed as a major flaw, an embarrassing enemy we must seek to destroy no matter what it takes. Even Billie Jean King is not immune. In a match in 1983, while still earning a living in sports after over twenty years and still a hero to millions of women, she constantly berated herself, bitterly repeating, "Get to the ball, fatso. C'mon, fatty, can't you run any faster than that." Even though her comments probably stemmed more from a desire for a better performance than from concerns about her appearance, it was still painful and humiliating to listen to one of my heroes abuse herself in such tones. Apparently, hating one's body if it is "too fat" is not limited to mere mortals but affects superstars as well.

Men and women educated in the highly competitive, no pain, no gain schools of physical education may be, ironically, the least well prepared to create a positive educational atmosphere for large women until they examine and change some of their own attitudes. A round table discussion among six top women athletes and fitness trainers, published in a 1987 edition of San Francisco's *City Sports* magazine, reveals much about why so many women are still inhibited from seeking fitness classes in the eighties. "Whenever there [are] men in the [aerobics] classes, the class is so much better. Because when some women get together, they often don't work hard enough. . . . [in] a beginning class, with just women, they have a social hour in there; they just talk and have a good time. And we need to say: 'C'mon, you guys, do something for your body, otherwise you're not going to get any results.' " From another woman in the discussion: "I think [women] come to my class even more than they go to your class because they can hide in the water. They're submerged, and nobody can look at them." Is it any wonder that many of us might be just a tad intimidated by such attitudes and choose to hide ourselves or not show up at all?

There has been great progress in improving access to sporting opportunities for women since the mid 1970s, from girls playing in Little Leagues to hundreds of thousands of dollars in athletic scholarships offered to women each year. But if the teachers who are supposedly tops in the fitness field (if you don't count actresses) are angry at women for not being as serious and results oriented as men, and if they criticize us for "inadequate efforts" and for laughing and enjoying ourselves, it's obvious that we still have a long way to go to make sport and fitness education more accessible to everyone.

In the view of Mary Boutilier and Lucinda San Giovanni in their marvelous book, *The Sporting Woman,* the standard emphasis of women's sports activists thus far—to seek equal access to the male-dominated sports establishment—is still too limited an approach to create concrete change. It has resulted in ". . . a general failure to extend the opportunities for women's sport participation to minority women, poor women, older women, lesbian women, fat women, working women, handicapped women—that is, to all those women who do not fit the model image of the 'promising athlete,' who may not be a good investment . . . or who want something different from what Sportsworld has traditionally offered. There has been a failure to seriously consider the range of alternative pathways for encouraging women to play sports. This has led to uncritical embracement of male-structured sports, with minor alterations, and wishful statements that 'we will be different.' " Rather than being different, many female physical educators have instead been co-opted by the values so fundamental to the institution of PE instruction. The vision of progressive women's sports educators like Boutillier and San Giovanni offers both hope and great illumination for setting a course of change, and their book is a must for anyone concerned with this issue.

We believe physical education teachers have an obligation to examine their attitudes because they are viewed by many as role models. They have skills and expertise the rest of us need. And in working with tenderhearted youth they can make or break an individual's desire and ability to continue physical activities into adulthood. But if they continue to foster a super-competitive, results oriented search for a "perfect body," then both children and adults will continue to be stymied in their search for a good education in physical movement. If you are a parent, do not hesitate to register your complaints if there is a PE instructor who you believe is undermining, rather than enhancing, your child's enjoyment of physical activity. An education in physical movement should inspire confidence and positive self-esteem, not create cringing memories of embarrassment and pain.

We also believe there is reason for large women to be cautiously optimistic. Many fitness instructors realize that they do not know firsthand about even the physical, let alone psychological, realities of living in a large body; therefore they must ask us what we need in order to design classes that will help us, not hinder us, in becoming more active. And many of them are asking. In some cities those instructors who are able to set aside any ulterior motive to whip us into "perfect" shape are being hired by groups of large women to teach classes sensitive to our needs. (We have included information in the appendix for those instructors interested in teaching classes designed with the safety and comfort of large women in mind.) We hope this infant trend will grow into lively adulthood.

Women, regardless of size, belong in the world of sport. In the words of Simone De Beauvoir, "Not to have confidence in one's body is to lose confidence in oneself. . . . It is precisely the female

athletes, who being positively interested in their own game, feel
themselves least handicapped in comparison with the male. Let
[women] swim, climb mountain peaks . . . take risks, go out for
adventure, and [they] will not feel before the world timidity." Sports
can be a way to learn about the marvels of our bodies and the joys
of recess but only if we know that we have choices. We can be
seriously competitive if we choose, can lighten up and just go for
enjoying ourselves, or maintain any attitude in between. There is no
"right" way to participate. We can also consciously choose to let any
unwarranted, uninvited, self-righteous criticism from any of the
super jocks and super bods simply dry up and blow away. We can
inhabit the world as strong women living with respect for ourselves
and our choices. We need not settle for less.

Choosing a Sporting Attitude

Neither the ability to play a sport nor the choice about what sport
you play is definitively linked to body size, although if you're seven
feet tall, you're more likely to be attracted to playing basketball than
becoming a jockey. Elite athletes use such physical characteristics as
muscle fiber types (slow-twitch versus fast-twitch) to determine
which bodies are better suited for short, intense sprints such as the
one-hundred-yard dash and which are suited for running one hundred miles. Such distinctions are irrelevant for the rest of us. If
enjoyment rather than winning first place is our goal, sport participation is far more dependent on developing an exploratory, curious
attitude than on determining which kind of muscle fibers we have.

The process of choosing a sport begins with basic desire. Once
that desire is firmly established—I want to play!—sensitive, knowledgeable instructors, proper equipment, reasonable goals, and enjoyable playing companions round out the process and make it fun.
Being open to trying different things may introduce you to sports
you never dreamed you could participate in.

This is not to say that a greater amount of weight does not
create greater challenge; your weight, particularly in combination
with any physical injury or limiting condition, may indeed influence
some of your activity choices. For instance, if you have a big belly
and a bad back, you're not likely to be attracted to rowing, but
swimming may fit the bill just fine. In my experience it is much easier
to backpack at 180 pounds than at 220, and at 250 I now take only
day hikes with a lightweight pack. But regardless of my size I always
enjoy outdoor adventures, am inspired by the gift of the wilderness,

and am empowered by the realization that I can do things I used to think were impossible. Very large women may never want to try sports that stress running, but they can become totally enthralled with water sports such as snorkling, scuba diving, and volleyball played in a pool.

While your weight may be one factor to consider when choosing sports activities, it is not the only one. The point is that you have a right to try any sport you want. Do not let other people's stereotypes or your own attitudes stand in your way. Get to know your own body, find an activity you like or think you'd like to try, and build up your strength gradually. The most important thing is to concentrate on your abilities, not your limitations.

But telling yourself to have a positive attitude is not enough. If you did not have a chance to run and play freely as a child, if you were intimidated by PE classes or ridiculed because of your "blubber," or if you simply haven't been interested in physical activity until now, you may live in a body that has not yet learned to love the feel of movement. This is understandable. It's natural to be concerned about the possibility of embarrassing or even injuring yourself as you huff and puff your way through some new activity. But these concerns will lessen as you gradually improve your aerobic conditioning, get to know and trust your body, learn skills in body awareness, gain support from other large women, and grow in confidence through experience.

Self-consciousness, self-doubt, and self-condemnation are strong emotions common to all adults trying to learn any new activity. These emotions are stumbling blocks even for elite athletes and may be so powerfully entrenched in your mind that even trying may seem too painful, too risky. Critical, self-doubting inner voices—How do I look? Am I doing it right? What do people think? How much farther?—can distract your attention and make it even more difficult for your body to move in ways that are natural and relaxed. But it can be done. Honest. Learning skills in relaxation, concentration, and visualization will help your mind, body, and emotions work together, and these skills will be discussed in Chapter 8. Giving yourself credit for the courage it takes to *try* is vital.

The human body is a marvelous creation that was meant to move and play, and this is true regardless of your body's size. Your body is an expert on movement, but too often a doubting, nagging, judgmental mind undermines the body and destroys its native confidence and competence. Learning how to short-circuit this destructive mental chatter is the key to restoring your body's self-confidence, and the skills stressed by sport psychologists will help you do this when you begin to try them. You'll be amazed how much your body can do once you get out of its way.

In addition, once you concentrate on the process and let go of the results, learning to appreciate and enjoy the present moment for what it is, a world of possibilities will open up to you. This is true not just of sports but of a wide range of endeavors. In essence, sports can be a training ground not only for your body but for your spirit. If you can take this emphasis on process rather than results into other areas of your life, too, you will find that you learn faster, enjoy more, and have less anxiety about any activity you choose.

Another attribute of a positive sporting attitude is its affirmation of play (or recess, as we keep calling it). This may feel a bit strange at first. As adults we often lose sight of the need for abandoning ourselves to playful, "irrelevant" activity. In the words of a typical Type A: "Playing is a waste of time. When you're done you have nothing to show for it." But too often heart attacks are what the super-competitive Type A's have to show for *their* efforts.

Bringing the spirit of play to any activity we try, we expand our capacity for enjoyment and our repertoire of pleasure. Both individual and team sports can be inspiring. Elite ability is not necessary to enjoy physical challenges. Winning is not the point; playing is. Build time into your day for fun as a special gift to yourself.

Pick a Sport, Any Sport

So what's your pleasure? Earlier you had a chance to think about what kind of activities you might enjoy. One thing to keep in mind when you are choosing a sport is that aerobic activities—such as walking, swimming, cycling—offer the most consistent benefit in improving heart and lung conditioning and overall fitness. Anaerobic (stop and go) kinds of activities—tennis, softball, volleyball, weight training—offer muscle toning, improvements in coordination, and the challenge of teamwork and/or competition. Both types of activities can be great fun.

Women who participate in various sports give a wide range of reasons for their choice. The idea of getting physically stronger, while perhaps foreign to many of us in the beginning, is in fact just what enticed weight lifter Taree Lyn Klausner to her sport in the first place. "I'm not doing this to lose weight—I'm getting bigger. And stronger. And it feels great! Being really strong has become a metaphor for my whole life. Whenever I'm in doubt I say to myself, 'If I lift weights as I do, I can certainly handle this.' "

Some women begin something new because their lives need a lift. Rita Northrop Jones says that before she began taking karate she was a little afraid of her body and spent her time indoors, waiting. "Waiting for what, I don't know, to die maybe. But then a karate studio opened up around the corner from my house, and one day I just got tired of waiting and went and joined. My daughter and I have been doing karate for four years now, and I feel like a totally new person, really alive and confident. I also kind of like showing the other people at the studio that a large woman can do just as much as anyone else."

If you want to try weight lifting or the martial arts, you'll need to do a little investigation to find a gym or class that meets your needs. Try to find out as much as you can about the sport before-

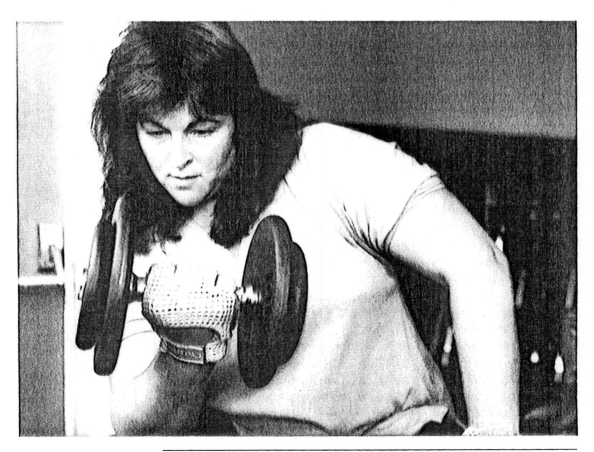

"Becoming stronger is a metaphor for my whole life," says Taree Lyn Klausner.

hand and don't take unnecessary risks. For instance, if you want to try weight lifting, get some instruction in a beginning Nautilus program at a gym rather than just charging in and hoisting bar bells. Remember to start slowly and build strength gradually. Read as much as you can get your hands on. If you are not lucky enough to live around the corner from a studio but decide you want to take a class or join a gym, don't rush out and join the first one you find in the Yellow Pages. Most classes and gyms offer a free introductory visit before you sign on the dotted line. I once went to a tai chi class expecting serene stretching and quiet concentration; I encountered a drill sergeant with a whistle around his neck. Needless to say I'm glad I didn't sign up for a six-week course before I had a chance to experience the class.

When choosing a gym, atmosphere is everything. You want to feel comfortable, not intimidated. You want the most value for your dollar. And you want the motto of "safety first" to be one the gym values as much as you do. Look for a family gym, which tends to be less competitive than singles gyms and usually offers separate areas for men and women. Some facilities have lap pools, and most offer weight rooms, stationary exercise bikes, and a variety of other equipment and classes. For pure comfort take a look at the showers, with bonus points given for saunas, whirlpools, or Jacuzzis. To fit gym time into your schedule, make sure the location and hours are convenient for you. And don't forget to ask about costs for bringing a guest and whether or not your membership can be transferred or held in waiting temporarily if you are ill, injured, or decide to move. If a club has been established only recently, look at the details that spell financial health so they don't decide to move some night and take your money with them. Details such as cleanliness, whether there are substitute instructors instead of cancelled classes, and even whether the toilet paper is in abundant supply can tell you a lot about financial stability or, conversely, whether they are trying to cut financial corners. Most important is the availability of qualified instructors who will help you develop an individualized program.

Starting with one activity and branching out to others, while certainly not necessary, is a very natural outcome of gaining confidence in your abilities. Linda Minor first became more physically active in an aerobics class called Light on Your Feet, designed for large women by Rosezella Canty-Letsome, and now also enjoys the pleasures of bicycling. "I really appreciate the conditioning benefits and the self-confidence bicycling gives me. I'm forty-two and my Dad is over seventy, and bicycling is the first thing we've ever been able to do together. It's great!" Michele Dethke incorporates many activities into her life—bicycling to work, spending one day each weekend on a longer bicycle adventure, and swimming and doing tai chi at other times in the week—proving once again that variety is the spice of life.

Cycling is good for aerobic conditioning and great for enjoyment, but it is not without risk. When thinking about cycling, many women fear ridicule more than injury. The fear of turning our backs (and our big behinds) to strangers and thus being vulnerable to any crude comments is one that can keep us immobile. But don't let the jerks of the world cheat you out of the joys of cycling. *Do,* however, pay heed to the very real potential danger of accidents.

A rude comment won't kill you. A skull fracture might. So buying a cycling helmet, usually at a cost of around $40 or so, is a very worthwhile investment and much cheaper than brain surgery. Fat tire "mountain bikes" allow you to venture onto dirt roads and trails, which can be safer than maneuvering through city traffic, particularly if bike lanes are not established where you live. (You could also lobby for some!) Regardless of the type of bike you buy, be sure it is the proper size for your height, and adjust the seat so that you get full extension of your legs while riding. Observing traffic rules and the safety tips outlined in any bike book should get you on your way to a healthy ride.

Some people prefer individual sports; others like the spirit and challenge of competition and may want to choose partner or team sports. Some, of course, mix and match. A woman joined a softball team I once played on just so we'd have enough players to enter the league, even though she thought she was "too fat to play" and would probably just watch. She ended up playing and loving it. Most of the team members were beginners, out mainly for fun, enticed by the idea of learning something new together. And there's just something thrilling about running out on a softball field in the spring with eight other people in matching shirts. After the first season, when we lost most of our games but still had a great time, this woman got into jogging to build up her strength and endurance so that two years later she was playing softball in the summer and soccer in the fall. You could never have told her in the beginning that she would eventually be organizing a coed soccer league just so she could learn it and play.

I learned to play softball at age thirty-four on a team with several American Indian women I worked with in a small rural town. Everyone in town played, it seemed—Little League teams for kids, serious interscholastic leagues for high school competitors, and many, many adult softball teams playing either fast-pitch or slow-pitch—so if you didn't play softball in the spring you felt you were missing all the fun. I had to learn all the basics from scratch—batting, throwing, and catching (but I staunchly refused to learn to slide into bases, figuring that was more of a commitment to risky adventure than I wanted to make)—and I had to master all the rules, too, so I wouldn't get hurt or make a fool of myself by running off the base at the wrong time.

Learning to play softball with Indian women had many advantages. A lot of them were great players and could give me excellent coaching and advice. Most important, though, in the context of this book, was the fact that many of them were also large women, and it was not considered at all unusual for them to be good players. Indians, in fact, had a reputation for being some of the best players, regardless of their size, since many of them had picked up their first bat and mitt when they were toddlers. Indian women showed me again and again that you did not have to be thin to be great at sports or to have a great time playing.

Even though I no longer play in a softball league, I love to go to the park and throw the ball around. Starting out slowly to warm up, it feels good to work up a rhythm, gradually throwing faster and harder. It's also fun to get up a game of adults and kids because then the focus really is on keeping the game fun for all, and there seems to be much more laughing as a result. This is the way many of you may get roped into your first game. There is nothing like kids saying, "C'mon, Mom, we just need one more player. All you have to do is stand there." Thanks for the vote of confidence, kids. Don't turn them down, though, because softball may be just your cup of tea. If you are interested in more serious fare, explore the league possibilities in your area.

Most team sports are organized in schools, by city recreation departments, or through work. You can either join an already existing team or form your own team and join a league. Probably the most important value to agree on when playing any team sport is whether the team is focused primarily on winning or on having fun and learning to play the game to everyone's best ability. Some teams love cutthroat competition, which is fine if everyone agrees on this value. Otherwise, there will be conflict. Once you feel confident you share the team's values, you can look forward to some good times. If you've never played on a team before, you will find it different from any individual sport you've engaged in. The telepathy that develops from practicing together and then making an outstanding play during a game is magic. Team spirit can be a very exhilarating feeling. Even consoling one another after a loss can be fun!

Some business management books say women are disadvantaged in the corporate world because we haven't learned teamwork on the playing field and therefore don't know what it's like to be part of a group working toward a common goal. This is ridiculous since women have natural skills and all kinds of experience in working together toward a common goal. How often have you seen a team of men put on a dinner for fifty people or set up a battered women's shelter with virtually no money? On the other hand, it is true that many women have not learned teamwork in the special context of playing sports. Without some experience in sports women may be unfamiliar with the metaphors that are used and with the underlying thrust of the football mentality that so dominates the corporate world. But more progressive management systems seem to be coming increasingly into vogue lately. With the high numbers of women who have entered the workforce in the last ten to fifteen years, some companies are beginning to recognize and value women's tendency toward a more cooperative, intuitive approach to problem solving. By the time our daughters arrive on the work scene they assuredly will have had the benefit of far more sporting opportunities than many of us had and hopefully will also find a corporate world far more appreciative of all their talents as well.

More Strenuous Stuff

We have written a great deal about taking your first safe steps toward a more active life and being gentle with yourself. This is not to say that as a larger woman you cannot participate safely in more strenuous activities if you wish. There is no reason to be afraid of injuring yourself in more strenuous activity if you prepare yourself.

Once you get well into a regular exercise program you may want to think about a more serious training routine and will need to know ways to increase your level of activity without increasing the possibility for injury. This process of seeing yourself "in training," while perhaps too jockish for some, may be just the incentive to prevent boredom for others. If you are a runner or cycler, you may want to train for a race. If you are a hiker, you may want to try backpacking. If you are a swimmer, you may want to try scuba diving. While there is no reason that you should set more strenuous goals if you enjoy your present routine, there is also no reason that you cannot set your sights on more difficult projects if you train for them properly.

One basic strategy of training is "hard . . . easy." In other words, you set up a routine that stretches your body's capacity for one exercise session and then take it easier the next session. Your body grows in muscle strength and cardiovascular endurance capacity by straining a bit and then resting. Your body needs both the increase in stress and the time to rest in order to get stronger. Recuperation time is a vital component of this process and one that is often ignored. Therefore, you can set up a schedule that will take recuperation time into account.

For instance, if you want to plan a backpacking trip and are walking for an hour a day, you could vary that time by adding an extra 30 to 60 minutes to your routine twice a week. Or you could begin to carry a ten- or fifteen-pound pack (books or bags of flour work fine) every other day you walk. If you do this, be sure you use a pack made for hiking so that the additional weight is distributed evenly. Once you get used to a particular amount of weight, you can increase it gradually if you wish. In this way your body will get used to carrying more weight and not go into shock if you put a forty-pound pack on your back and try to walk uphill!

There are many books to use as guidelines to develop a training routine just right for the particular activity you choose, and we have included some suggestions in the bibliography. Once you get interested in a greater variety of activities, your library of exercise books will probably increase in direct proportion to your enthusiasm. While your body may be larger than the one most authors have in mind when they write their books, there is no reason you cannot safely adapt some of their ideas and principles to your own needs. Good books will outline specific training routines to increase your strength and abilities gradually, and exercise routines will vary depending on the particular kind of activity.

The reason we have mentioned the idea of more strenuous exercise is to encourage you to decide to do what *you* want to do and not settle for less. You don't necessarily have to avoid more strenuous exercise because of your weight. If you train for a goal by using a hard-easy mode, listen to your body as you go, and get proper information and help when you need it, there is no reason why you cannot try for exactly what you want. There is no way to know your full potential when you begin. You may surprise yourself over and over.

* * *

There are some sports that are aerobic, offering a full body workout without high impact or stress on joints—swimming, skating, hiking, rowing, canoeing, cross-country skiing, and cycling are such sports. Other sports, while not aerobic, still offer the pleasure of a sporting experience—challenging yourself, learning a skill, developing awareness of your body in motion, sharpening your reflexes, improving your physical performance, gaining in self-confidence, and experiencing the exhiliration of accomplishment. Archery, golf, bowling, table tennis, fencing, sailing, and frisbee are such sports, and ones that you might also like to try. You need not limit yourself to just those sports from which you're likely to get the most health benefits, although this might be one important criterion for selection at first. But remember that there is fun to be had in lots of different activities, and just because you've never tried them until now doesn't mean you never will. Sports are for every body. Yours too.

In the words of distance swimmer Diana Nyad, speaking to the 1983 New Agenda Conference of athletes, coaches, and educators charting the future of women in sport: "I stand here before you feeling like I own the earth because of 20 years in a sport. That's what we're fighting for—to make sure that everybody out there, every little girl and every high school girl and every 55-year-old woman ashamed of her fat could feel like I feel—like she owns the earth."

Maybe someday there will be no girl or woman ashamed of her fat and we will all feel like we own the earth on which we stand. It seems like a worthy goal toward which to work.

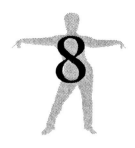

Learning
Body Awareness

Tips from Sport Psychology

I was the fattest person in the room. The only fat person, actually. (I have always noticed my fat ranking, ever since third grade when the nurse began to weigh us every year and hollered out the amount for a secretary to write down. Every year I was third fattest in my class.) This time the classroom was filled with jocks; it was my first sport psychology course, and I kept trying to hide my belly.

The instructor said we were to share a "peak experience" in sport. Great. Oh, I'd had peak experiences all right, those moments of exhilarating clarity: running my first race and finishing about three feet off the ground in my excitement; catching an impossible fly in center field; hiking to the top of a waterfall I had previously only squinted at from a distant position far below. But considering there were college athletic coaches and even a former pro basketball player in the room, let's just say I felt distinctly out of my league. The first student to speak told a hair-raising story of "extreme skiing" off cliffs in Switzerland. Uh-oh. Sure, I could tell myself that my story was fine and that I shouldn't compare myself with others, but I compared anyway. My stories would seem embarrassingly tame, even sedentary, to these folks, I thought. I had quit my job, moved four hundred miles across the state, and this was the first class in a graduate school program I'd dreamed about for many years. I left the class wondering if I could get my old job back. By the time I arrived home I dissolved in despair. What made me think I could do this? Maybe I should just give up and get some exercise by running away.

After spending fifteen years in a reclining position, when I became reactivated at thirty-one it was through yoga and playing tennis. Until that time I'd gotten by on my brains and bravado, and treated my body as if somehow "it" was dispensable and "I" could go on just fine without it. If you'd said "body awareness" to me then, I would have said: "Who wants to be aware of this!" I hated my body and was not interested in being any more aware of it than necessary.

Through yoga I began to come home to my body. I learned the slow, concentrated movements and to use my breath to help me extend in the direction I was stretching and not worry about whether I reached a specific destination. I learned what my body felt like on the inside when it moved and became gradually less concerned with what it looked like on the outside. When I began, sitting on the floor with my legs outstretched, I couldn't even come close to touching my toes. After a month of almost daily practice, I could touch my face to my knees and wrap my hands around my feet. I'd always thought I was inflexible. So much for accurate perceptions about my potential. Anything seemed possible after that. Tiny seeds of self-acceptance were firmly planted.

Through tennis, practicing some of the focusing and awareness techniques of the Inner Game that are introduced in this chapter, I found another fascinating way to become more comfortable in my body, this time during more vigorous movement. Around this time I also began formulating plans for the graduate school program that a few years later landed me in the fateful first class with the jocks. What I'd learned in yoga and tennis had helped me heal some of the wounds fat-hating had created. After graduation I planned to use my experience to help other women learn to become more comfortable in their bodies too. Who knows, I might even find a way to become lastingly thin, I thought, although I'd practically given up that idea after five years of running hadn't budged my weight below 185. But you'll notice I said "practically," which of course is why I felt so vulnerable in the class as I unconsciously began to compare myself to the elite athletes. The seeds of self-acceptance I'd been nurturing through the years had certainly helped me grow stronger and were some of the reasons I had gotten to graduate school in the first place. But once there I felt that again my fat body had betrayed me.

Fortunately, a friend helped me realize that it was my attitude, not my body, that had betrayed me.

With her help I remembered that whenever I compared myself to others I always found someone thinner, smarter, faster, or better at an activity than I was. So why put myself through that? It's not third grade anymore. I could simply be me now, and it was enough. But old habits are hard to break, and new ideas take seemingly endless practice to replace them. I'd prepared myself, and I believed I had a right to be in that class—it was a public university and I'd paid my money! But regardless of all my preparation, when I arrived at the moment of truth all of my internalized fears about fat women not *really* belonging in sport surfaced. It wasn't as if someone in the room stood up and pointed at me and my belly and said: "Hey you, fat one, *out!*" What did happen was that I rejected myself before someone else got the chance. *My* critical voice tried to exclude me and keep me from my dream, not a critical voice from that classroom. And it was my self-critical voice that I could change.

The world may say I'm inappropriate for sport because I'm fat, but I don't have to believe it. Changing my attitude doesn't change the world, to be sure; prejudice does exist. But changing my self-critical attitude does keep me from making matters worse for myself. If I just remember to stay focused on reaching in the direction of my dream, breathe, relax, and stick to it, I will become stronger and more flexible, and can surpass what I think is not possible in the beginning.

I believed in my own experience; I knew of the healing potential of body awareness and sport psychology. So I went back, and the class turned out to be one of the most enjoyable I've ever taken.

Many discussions centered around how we could coach ourselves and others into more confident, self-aware ways of playing, and some of those ideas are included here. All talk was not just about "peak experiences" and glowing reports of success, however. We also talked about our most embarrassing moments, which everyone had also experienced, even the most accomplished athletes. All of the discussions strengthened my view that the techniques we were discussing could work just as well for beginners and the "non-elite" as they do for the most highly skilled athlete. And when the former pro basketball player turned out to be one of the most low-key, understanding people in the class instead of a hyper-competitive lout, as many jocks are stereotyped, it became obvious once more just how ridiculous and damaging all stereotyping is. It works to keep people alienated from one another and off balance. And it is totally unnecessary.

I also learned that even when I feel out of place at first, I usually have a lot more in common with other people than any surface appearance can predict initially. If I stay with a situation, it soon becomes more comfortable. If it doesn't, there is always plenty of time to leave once I have given myself a chance. In this instance, I'm sure glad I didn't run away.

If the world of sport psychology seems a distance from where you are now, it may be because it is so routinely associated with elite athletes that you feel awkward even considering it. But I hope my experience is helpful to you. If you compare yourself to elite athletes, surely you will lose. Comparison is both unnecessary and counter-productive. If you can let go of any stereotype you may have about how "inappropriate" it is that you are trying to learn these skills and just try to take things one step at a time and give yourself a chance, you will begin to marvel at how much your body can actually do. Learning the skills of concentration, relaxation, and visualization provides a way to shift your attention and your attitude away from self-criticism toward self-awareness and discovery. This shift can be, I believe, most liberating in the search for self-acceptance. It certainly helps me when I take my own advice.

Tips from the World of Sport Psychology

She bounced up and down on her skis at the starting gate, psyching herself up for a run at the 1984 Olympic gold medal in the women's slalom. "Just have fun . . . have fun . . . *have fun!*" she chanted. At the start signal, she shot out of the gate and down the mountain into the history books. Our skiing friend certainly needed more than her fun chant to have a crack at a gold medal—it also took Olympic-level ability, years of practice, and enough money for equipment, travel, and professional coaching. But on that most important day she used the mental focus of the chant to inspire her "go for it" self and override any nervousness, worry, or self-doubt that could have blocked her natural talents. Not only did she win the race but, you could tell when watching her ski, she really was having fun!

Elite athletes are the beneficiaries of the very best that sport science and coaching have to offer. Most of us are not, but it's never too late to learn to be your own coach. Much of this chapter is concerned with helping you do just that.

Sport psychology is a relatively new chapter in the athletic coach's playbook. It is used to help motivate athletes and improve their performance. Athletes learn to relax, to concentrate totally in the moment of play, and to use mental images to achieve their goals. With a tone of reverence and conviction formerly reserved for running thousands of conditioning miles or doing hundreds of sit-ups a day, athletes talk about how they've learned to use mental concentration and positive thinking to improve both their performance and their enjoyment of the sport.

The purpose of these techniques is to maximize your body's natural ability and minimize what gets in the way of that. By eliminating anxious or self-critical inner voices you *allow* rather than force your body to reach its potential. If our skiing friend allowed destructive mental chatter—I can't do it. Everyone else went so fast. I wonder how icy that turn at gate 16 is—to get in her way, she might not have done so well and certainly wouldn't have enjoyed her run so much. It is not always the most physically gifted athlete who wins the medal, then, but the athlete who can also trust herself, clear her mind of distractions, and become totally involved in the present moment. Her body knows how to ski. If her mind can focus on fun, allowing her body to stay loose and relaxed in the process, she can ski her best.

If when you go to a dance class you are constantly worrying—I'm too fat, too clumsy to do this. Everyone else seems so good at it and must think I'm gross. I'll never be able to do those leg lifts we do at the end of the class—you'll never know how well your body might function if you were concentrating only on learning to exhale at exactly the same moment during each leg lift. While your body is in motion you can visualize your muscles working smoothly and becoming stronger rather than criticize yourself for being a "weakling" because you may not be going as fast as others around you. Fear and doubt create muscle tension, and tense muscles simply will not perform as smoothly as relaxed ones. In addition, tense muscles are most vulnerable to injury. The trick is to focus on learning what to do *instead* of gritting your teeth and listening to demoralizing mental chatter.

In the words of a 1986 World Series game-winning home run hitter, "Concentration is the ability to think of absolutely nothing at the moment that it counts the most." The ability to stop destructive and distracting mental chatter and concentrate completely on what you're doing in the heat of the moment—whether at bat or on the dance floor—is a skill that can be learned. You can practice during movement and then apply it throughout your life (to calm your nerves just before an important job interview, for instance). It is not my intention, nor is it possible here, to give you more than a rudimentary introduction to a few sport psychology concepts. I'd simply like to whet your curiosity with some approaches you may not have tried yet. If you then want to pursue any of these ideas further, there are many books that can give you more information, including a few suggestions in the bibliography.

Learning the Inner Game

If you are not sure what I mean when I talk about this whining, carping inner voice, drift by a tennis court some day. It's amazing to hear the savage mutterings, name-calling, and put-downs that people address to *themselves* while trying to play. And people do this for fun? For health? Seems like a leisurely stroll at the beach would be better for the psyche than five minutes of this kind of self-criticism. And yet, on any given day, on any tennis court, you can find those mutterers. I know, I used to be one.

I started taking tennis lessons when I was six, playing in tournaments at the end of the summer every year. As I got older I began to live with a monster in my head. Every time I missed a shot, the monster would snicker and say, "See, hotshot, you missed another one. Some tennis player." I'd get angry and more frustrated at every shot I missed until I was so upset that I'd burst out with a string of names for myself. I'd end up furious—for looking bad, for losing, and then, given my outburst, for making a fool of myself. Even when I didn't have outbursts, I'd carry around this judge in my head who watched my every move, quick to criticize even minute failings and blow them all out of proportion. It seemed no matter how well I played, the monster was never satisfied.

After a fifteen-year hiatus from tennis I began playing again at age thirty-one and became fascinated with the approach introduced by Tim Gallwey in 1974 in his book, *The Inner Game of Tennis* (see Appendix). The inner game applies Eastern meditation techniques, similar to those used in yoga or Zen meditation, to this thoroughly Western sport. Gallwey explored the idea of Self-One and Self-Two, athletes with distinctly different characteristics living inside each of us. Self-One is the ever critical judge that keeps up the mental chatter that gets in our way. (Aha, he knew about my monster!) Self-Two is our natural body, our natural talent for movement that flourishes when the judgmental voice of Self-One is silenced. The trick, according to Gallwey, is to engage the critical or fearful Self-One in very specific activities that will then allow Self-Two, the natural player, to play well, unencumbered by criticism or doubt.

Gallwey's book introduced me to an entire array of things to do *instead* of letting the monster run wild in my brain. Most important, it helped me learn how to stay in the present and to enjoy the process of playing and not get hung up on the outcome of the game. Rather than beginning a game thinking, "Oh damn, my backhand has been so lousy, I can't hit those high, bouncing, top spin shots, and even if I could, it's no fun. I'll just lose this game; then I'll be down two and will never come back and will make a fool of myself. Oh why did I think I wanted to play this game anyway," I used Gallwey's tricks to engage my mind monster's attention elsewhere.

One exercise he suggested was simple: Watch the seams of the tennis ball as it approaches. Next to "bend your knees," the most common refrain from sport instructors is "watch the ball." In tennis I'd look at the ball, of course, but somehow I'd often hit it poorly, and the monster would have a field day. By focusing my attention even more narrowly—first on the seams of the ball, then on the

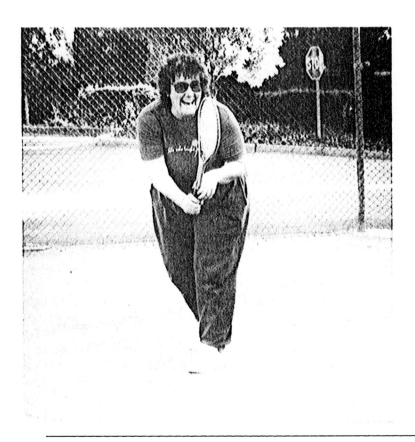

She who laughs lasts, especially while learning the "inner game" of tennis.

direction the ball was spinning as it came toward me—I found that my concentration was entirely consumed by the task at hand, with none left over for worry about the score, the future, or whatever. Another exercise involved tuning in to my breathing and then trying to stroke the ball on an exhale every time. Just by becoming aware of it, not even trying to change, I felt my breathing become more relaxed. And timing my strokes to my breathing made them more relaxed, too, as well as more effective.

The Bounce-Hit game was another favorite technique. The point of this game is to say "bounce" at the exact moment when the ball bounces on either side of the court and "hit" at the exact moment contact is made between racket and ball. This simple bounce-hit exercise gave my Self-One something tangible to do instead of ragging on me. "Bounce-hit, bounce-hit" apparently takes the place of "you jerk, you jerk." Meanwhile, my Self-Two could become absorbed in the rhythm of the play in the exact moment of the ball's contact with the court surface and either my or my partner's racket. With my attention totally focused on the ball, I could therefore "see" it better and thus hit it more often, which is of course the point of the game. My attention became drawn to observing closely how and where the ball was bouncing, which then almost magically resulted in my hitting the ball in the center of the racket strings much more frequently. Not only was it a relief to rid myself of the mental monster and critical judge, but I played much better and, not surprisingly, had more fun.

It is this focus in the bounce-hit present moment that prevents you from getting lost in recriminations about past failures or anxiety about future ones. Staying in the present allows Self-Two, your confident inner athlete, to take over and do what it knows how to do.

To learn to let go of fear and critical judgments is to learn to allow yourself to play your best. This is true in life as well as in tennis. You *cannot* deal now with the millions of potential problems that could arise in the future or did arise in the past; you *can* learn to deal with what is actually occurring. All any of us can really do is learn to stay in the present.

Learning to stay in the moment is a combination of distracting your critical mind and increasing your awareness of "what is." Increasing your awareness involves learning to focus your attention not only on exactly what is happening outside of you but what is happening inside as well—your breathing, muscle tension, joint flexibility, and balance. Awareness is observation, curiosity, watching; it is not judgment. Gallwey's books on inner tennis, and *Inner Skiing* written with Bob Kriegel, explore many ways to learn awareness of "what is" during these two sports. Their ideas can be adapted to virtually any activity you might choose if you'd like to pursue them further.

In principle, what they point out is that heightened concentration on the details of the present automatically diverts your attention from any doubting or critical mental chatter and also gives you information you may not have had before. Learning self-awareness is a step-by-step process that is as crucial to improving your self-esteem as it is to developing the confidence you need to take physical risks. But it takes time. Awareness does not come overnight. If you have not devoted sufficient time to heightening your awareness of your body in motion, it is most likely because you have not been encouraged to do so.

It is not surprising that Gallwey's adaptation of Eastern movement philosophies can be so successful for those of us looking for a different way to approach the so thoroughly Western world of sports. The competitive, individualistic nature of our society has convinced us that in order to achieve success we must do it on our own and that our success must come by winning over others. Our attention is often focused outside ourselves, on comparisons with our "competition," rather than inside ourselves on our own development.

In Gallwey's view, focusing on our competition is highly likely to limit us. In addition, it is often the focus on *trying* itself, particularly if we are trying *hard,* that is least likely to be helpful no matter what we're doing. Close your eyes for a moment and get an image in your mind of a teacher saying, "Try harder. Harder! Concentrate!" Can't you feel your stomach churn? Your muscles tense? Maybe you even unconsciously clenched your fist in anger at the suggestion that you were not trying hard enough the first time. How can this possibly help us concentrate, let alone improve our performance? Creating tension, either muscle or emotional tension, improves neither our concentration nor our performance, and certainly it doesn't improve our enjoyment either. If our goal is to allow our mind, body, and emotions to work together, then we must develop skills that promote more balance and harmony.

It's also well to keep in mind that sports often overemphasize the development of the muscles in one part of the body, while less attention is given to the body overall. For instance, racket and bat-and-ball sports involve using primarily one side of the body or the other, such as in batting right-handed. While running strengthens the muscles of the legs, it does very little for the upper body.

Most sports also emphasize lots of muscle contractions, but do not allow equal time for muscle relaxation and stretching. Western sports often place so much value on developing hard muscles that we might lose sight of the fact that strength and competence need not come from muscle power alone.

In contrast, Eastern movement disciplines such as yoga, tai-chi, karate, and aikido, while very different in appearance and practice, all share the central idea that energy (called *Ki* by the Japanese) flows throughout the body and that strength, balance, and competence come from focusing this energy. If one is not in balance, energy is blocked and thus so is strength and coordination. The physical focus of these movement disciplines always includes breathing and seeking balance during a variety of movements that utilize virtually all of the body's muscle groups. The mental focus is on heightening one's awareness of internal energy flow. The center of the internal energy system is the midpoint of the abdomen, which means that movements that flow outward from this center are more likely to be movements full of strength and balance.

You can get a sense of the difference between muscle strength and strength generated by heightened concentration on energy flow by trying two experiments. Choose a partner of about equal strength. Make a fist and stand with one of your arms outstretched in front of you, straight from your shoulder. If you are right-handed, use your right arm since it is likely to be your stronger arm. Your partner will place her hands on your outstretched fist and *gradually* use all of her strength to press your arm downward while you try to resist with all the muscle strength you can muster. Pretend you're Superwoman. Tighten your fist and all the muscles in your straightened arm. (You can even tighten your other fist and grit your teeth if you want to get the sense of really trying hard.) When you're ready, give your partner the signal to begin. Resist with all your strength. Come on, try hard! Pay attention to how your body feels while you're trying to resist. When you're finished, shake your arm out to release any tension that tightening your muscles created before starting the next experiment.

This time your partner will try the same method of pressing your arm downward, but you'll use a different method to resist. Place your feet about one to one and one half feet apart on the floor so that you feel comfortably and firmly planted. Take a deep breath and bend your knees slightly. Don't lock them. Feel the floor beneath your feet and know that underneath the floor, some layers below, is good old Mother Earth. Now close your eyes for a moment and imagine that a beam of light has come up through the floor from the earth, entering your body through your feet and gradually flowing up your legs and throughout your entire body. See this beam of light get brighter and stronger with each breath; the brightest spot is in the center of your abdomen. Stretch your arm straight out in front of you again. This time, instead of clenching your fist and tightening all your muscles, keep your outstretched arm straight but totally relaxed. Wiggle your fingers to be sure they are loose. Keep your attention on the light flowing throughout your body. The light gives your arm rock-solid firmness. Do not hold your breath. Allow relaxed breathing to strengthen the constant flow of light as it comes from deep in the earth and flows throughout your body, particularly as it strengthens your arm. When you have this image firmly in place, signal your partner to try to press your arm downward again as you keep breathing. Again, notice how your body feels this time while you try to resist.

What differences did you find in the two experiences? In doing this exercise with many different groups over the years, I've found that most people are amazed at how much stronger they are with the imagery created in the second attempt than when they try to use muscle strength. By keeping your attention focused on the constant flow of energy, more energy is generated. In addition, while the first session of trying hard is more likely to increase tension, people relate feelings of calm generated by the second experience. This is not surprising since concentrating on the internal energy flow is a way to tune in to the harmony of the universe and its energy flow.

Learning to focus on your internal energy is a way to experience your body in a new way—from the inside out. It is a way to affirm the fact that you need not be all hard muscle in order to be strong. Furthermore, centering activities of breathing and focusing promote relaxation and thus are great for stress reduction. By learning to place the bulk of your effort in actions that heighten your own awareness of "what is," and to become more adept at focusing on your internal energy flow, you are much less likely to get caught in the comparison-to-other-players trap so common to athletics. If you are interested in learning more about any of the Eastern movement disciplines or martial arts, look for classes in your area. Either alone or in combination with sports, these activities are both fascinating and full of rich learning potential.

It is one thing to focus on our breathing and internal awareness while we are standing still or doing a short exercise. It is quite another to learn to focus our awareness internally when we are in motion for much longer periods of time, particularly if it is a motion that we have come to take for granted, such as walking. It takes practice. Try the next exercise for a little practice.

Walking with Awareness

"Stand up straight," my mother used to say because I had a tendency to walk slouched over and round shouldered. As one of the first girls in my fourth-grade class to have to wear a bra, I tried to hide my chest to avoid snide comments from the boys, which of course didn't work anyway. As I got a little older, the command from the world was, "Suck in your stomach," and when natural sucking methods didn't work, I started wearing a girdle, which damaged my circulation to say nothing of the discomfort involved in being stuffed into a piece of rubber. Instead of developing a natural pride in my body and a free, relaxed walking stride to match, I became more and more self-conscious about how I looked and unconscious of how I actually moved. For me, part of the process of becoming more active included relearning how my body actually felt when I moved, particularly how it felt when I moved in a more balanced way. I've been practicing a more internal focus for years and am still learning.

The following exercise will give you a brief introduction to becoming more attuned to your body in motion. While you are walking you will shift your internal focus from one part of your body to another for about twenty minutes overall. As in Chapter 2 you may want to have a partner read the exercise to you, or you may want to tape it and play it back. Or you may be able to just read it through, try it, and then reread it to see if you caught all the steps. At first it may be difficult for you to isolate individual muscle groups, but this will get much easier with practice. Learning the ability to concentrate on one part of your body will help enhance the performance of the movement and minimize the potential for injury in that particular muscle group as well as increase your overall body awareness.

Before you get started, think for a moment about your breathing. Exercise instructors frequently chirp, "Don't forget to breathe!" Well, it may sound stupid, but it's very common to hold your breath unconsciously or to breathe very shallowly. You may have noticed that you held your breath in the first experiment above when you were using muscle strength alone. Unconsciously holding your breath can happen whether you're watching TV or doing sit-ups, but when you're doing sit-ups your muscles need oxygen to move smoothly and efficiently. Holding your breath can create muscle tension when cells become starved for oxygen. And we've already seen how muscle tension can undermine performance. Learning how you breathe at rest and then practicing deep, full breathing are the first steps in building your internal awareness and promoting relaxed movement. You may want to return at this point to the relaxation exercise in Chapter 2 to help you remember how your body feels when it is relaxed and when you are deep breathing at rest. It will give you a point of comparison once you get into motion.

Find a place to do this exercise where you can walk around with some freedom and not have to worry about bumping into things. If your home is large enough, it's easiest to start there, back and forth in your living room, or perhaps try using your yard. If this is not possible, find a local park or even a sidewalk in your neighborhood, somewhere you do not have to deal with traffic. Your attention will be focused inward while you are walking, so this exercise is best done where you can control external hazards because awareness won't do you much good if you're run over by a bus in the process.

Begin by slowly walking around as you normally do. Don't do anything special. The point is to get your body moving just the way it always does. Do this for at least a minute and notice how your body is feeling.

Now stand in one spot, close your eyes, and take three or four deep, cleansing breaths. Feel any tension drain out of your body as you exhale. Begin to lift your heels off the ground slightly and start "walking" again but in place this time. Notice how the bottoms of your heels feel when they touch the ground. If there is any tension in your ankles as you move your heels up and down, allow your breath to release it when you exhale. After walking in place a few moments, open your eyes and begin walking forward slowly. Keep your vision sort of fuzzy and unfocused so that instead of looking all around you keep your attention internal and use your vision only to keep from bumping into objects.

Notice how your feet meet the earth from your heel all the way to the end of your toes. Spread your toes slightly for a few steps. Notice the length of your stride.

A few moments later, focus your attention on the muscles in your calves. Notice if there is any discomfort when these muscles contract. After a few moments, allow your focus to rise to your knees. Visualize your knees initiating your steps instead of your feet. See if you can get a sense of exactly how much your knees are bending with each step even if it is only slightly. Notice whether both knees seem to bend about the same amount. Walk this way for a little while, then pick up your pace. Notice if your knees are bending more now that you are going a bit faster. Notice the length of your stride at this increased pace. After a few moments, gradually slow your pace again.

Let your focus rise to the muscles in the front of your thighs. Continue to "lead" your walking motion with your knees but now with the added focus of your thigh muscles providing your knees with more stability.

After a few minutes, let your focus rise to the small of your back. Notice how the muscles there move with each step. Is there any feeling of tension or discomfort? If there is, take a deep breath and allow the tension to leave your body when you exhale. Repeat the deep breaths a couple of times.

Let your focus rise again to your upper back and your shoulders. Notice the movement in your shoulders as you swing your arms. Notice whether both arms are moving the same distance in front and behind your torso as you walk. Let them swing in this balanced way if you like. Is there any tension in your shoulders or your arms as you move along? If so, circle your shoulders forward a few times, then reverse. Stay with your attention in your shoulders for a little longer.

Let your attention focus on your head and neck. Gently turn your head from side to side. Allow your breath to release any tension in your neck. Let your jaw relax.

After a few moments, allow your attention to rest in the center of your chest. Take some slow, deep breaths, filling your lungs with the fresh air around you. Lift your rib cage slightly as you inhale. Feel the wind flow completely through your abdomen as your rib cage rises and falls. Continue this a few minutes.

Finally, allow your attention to center in the middle of your abdomen. Feel your abdomen fill with warmth and light as your attention rests there. While you keep walking, see a beam of light flow outward from your abdomen, leading you along. Walk this way for a few minutes. Then gradually slow your pace until you wish to stop.

After you have come to a stop, close your eyes and allow your attention to remain in your abdomen for a few moments more. Luxuriate in the warmth your muscles generated while walking. Let a few deep breaths enhance the flow of warmth throughout your body. When you are ready the exercise is over.

Most of us are oblivious to all of the coordinated muscle action necessary to move our bodies from place to place. This exercise helps heighten your awareness of how all the muscles in your body, not just those in your legs and feet, work together to accomplish the task of walking. This exercise was geared to include a total body focus. However, it is probably more effective to choose one particular muscle group or body location to focus on and stay with it throughout one walking experience. It is particularly effective if you experience any discomfort in a particular location such as your knees. If you focus your attention on just how your knees are feeling while you walk and then expand your focus to include your quadriceps (the muscles in the front of the thighs) chances are you will learn much about what may be creating the discomfort. If you alter the length of your stride, it might reduce the discomfort. If you exaggerate the bend in your knees with each step, it may give you even more information. Experiment. You have all the "laboratory" time you wish to take.

Oftentimes, by simply heightening your conscious awareness of a movement you allow Self-Two to lead your body into a better state of balance. This is important because if an imbalance does occur at some point (due, perhaps, to an injury or the development of poor posture habits), other muscles try to compensate and adjust so that you can keep going. The weakened muscles can become more and more dependent on the overcompensating ones so that the resulting exacerbation of the imbalance sends your muscles into spasm, which can be very painful. Even if you get by in relative comfort while in a state of imbalance, as many people do, any increase in your activity, say from walking to running, can produce pain or contribute to an injury. Once again, becoming aware of just how your body moves may be your best insurance against injury.

The ability to engage your full attention on specific body parts can also be an antidote to the boredom or distraction that may set in during your regular exercise activity. And if you're concentrating on visualizing your quadriceps as sturdily leading your motion, you will be far less concerned with "how much farther." Concentrating on keeping the amount of bend in each knee equal will keep your overall step much more balanced. And if you keep reminding yourself to breathe, maybe even timing your exhalations to match every third time your right foot hits the ground, for instance, you can establish a more regular rhythm.

The most important thing to remember about doing these activities is that they are learning activities, not exercises in self-criticism. You are learning to *quiet* the Self-One judge and let Self-Two curiosity dominate your attention. But it takes practice and patience to do this because you can't reverse a lifetime of negative

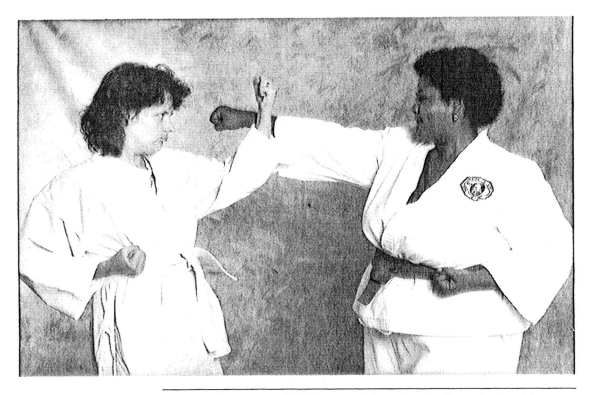

Karate combines strength, balance, and determination for enthusiasts Margaret
Orlando and Rita Northrop Jones.

programming overnight. And even after years of practice I still
struggle with the Self-One judge. It is far, far quieter now, but when
I least expect it—such as on the first day of my sport psychology
class, for instance—it springs into action. Tenacity seems to be one
of its main characteristics, so I just have to keep practicing.

By developing an appreciation for the marvel your body already
is—breath, bones, brains, blood, muscles, nerves, tendons and, yes,
even fat, working together in harmony—you can gradually improve
your body image, self-esteem, and self-confidence. None of us is
meant to live from the chin up. We are whole people and can coax
ourselves toward greater harmony. We can begin to act with more
power to be ourselves based on strength and energy flowing from
within. And we can appreciate our softness as well. We need not
become "hard bodies" to gain self-respect. Take a deep breath and
begin your internal journey fueled by curiosity, not judgments.

Mental Movies, You're the Star

Visualization is another technique that can be learned and used in a variety of situations. It is one more way to help your mind and body learn to work more effectively together. Essentially, visualization or imaging is a specific technique to produce a mental movie in which you watch yourself achieving what you want. It's more than simple daydreaming because you consciously induce a state of relaxation through breathing and help your mind and body work together.

Have you heard of self-fulfilling prophecies? Usually they are in the context of failure—you go to a job interview with the idea that you don't deserve the job and, sure enough, you don't get it. But visualization takes the idea of self-fulfilling prophecies and puts it to work toward positive outcomes. For instance, before going to the job interview you visualize successfully interviewing for the job and accepting the position when it is offered. Athletes such as the skier we met earlier do visualization exercises for several weeks before a race to "see" themselves skiing successfully around every flag on the course and crossing the finish line in record time. It is said the most successful athletes are often those who practice visualizing themselves making the moves they want in crucial situations. They are not born with the knowledge of visualization but have learned it. You can too.

Why should I want to, you say. First, it is an easy, inexpensive, and effective way to train. For instance, you can become a more relaxed and powerful swimmer through visualization. Researchers have found that when you get good at achieving a state of relaxation and visualizing your muscles working in unison, your muscle fibers actually twitch in response to the mental picture being created. You can, in effect, practice swimming out of the water. Although there is no aerobic benefit (sorry), positive muscle patterns can be strengthened through this mental practice.

It is helpful to watch someone who is good at the activity you want to try in order to get a clear picture in your mind. Then it will be a matter of seeing yourself moving just that way. Watching others play a sport is extremely helpful in forming the vision you want for yourself, particularly if you are a beginner and don't quite know exactly how the movements are supposed to look. Remember, you don't have to aspire to be a great athlete to get benefit from watching one. You don't have to do it exactly as they do, but you can adapt their movements to your mental picture of yourself. (Don't get caught up in comparing your body or your ability to theirs, though; just be curious and observe.) It is most helpful to do the visualization exercise just before you do your activity—get the strong mental picture and then put it into action—but certainly you can do it at any time.

The second reason you might want to learn this technique is that it is a way to get in touch with your inner self and learn more about how your mind and body can work together effectively. It's a way to quiet any useless or distracting mental chatter and put positive images in place instead. The third and most important reason is that it is an enjoyable way to take time for yourself.

Allow about 15 minutes for the next exercise. Find a comfortable place to lie down and relax. Decide what image you want to project on your mental movie screen. For the purposes of this exercise I've used swimming as the activity, but you can visualize anything you want once you learn the technique.

Lie on your back in the most comfortable position possible, knees bent or a pillow beneath them if that feels best. Allow your arms to relax at your sides. Begin to breath slowly, deeply, and relaxed. Inhale through your nose and exhale through your mouth. Simply allow your breathing to become more and more relaxed for a few moments. Let any distracting thoughts drift through your mind until they dissolve.

Count backwards from ten, allowing your body to relax more deeply with each count. By the time you reach one you will be very relaxed. With your eyes closed, get a picture in your mind of your body lying there very relaxed, breathing deeply.

Gradually form a picture of yourself standing at the edge of a large, spacious swimming pool. It is uncrowded and inviting. Get a clear picture of the color and pattern of your swimsuit. Hear any noises being made by the other swimmers. Anticipate that the water will be warm and welcoming when you enter.

See yourself enter the water, going down the steps one by one. While gliding slowly down the steps, experience how good the warm water feels on your skin. Try to get as clear a sense of how the water feels as possible. Walk in the water for a few moments, starting at the shallow end of the pool and working your way to deeper water. Feel the sensuous warmth of the water move up your body. See your goggles in place, ready to swim.

See yourself begin a gentle breaststroke with your head out of the water and your arms and legs moving in rhythm. After a few strokes put your face in the water and see how clear the water looks and the lines on the bottom of the pool. The voices of the other swimmers are lost in the calm silence of this underwater world you are in now. Continue to see yourself exploring the water for a few laps with this slow, gentle breaststroke. Feel the tension draining from your body with the gradual full body stretching this stroke involves.

In your mind's eye roll over on your back and begin to do the backstroke. Feel the muscles in your shoulders, back, and chest move with each stroke, allowing your chest to open up more fully. See your stroke become gradually more powerful as you glide through the water. Feel your legs kicking rhythmically but not creating a big splash.

See yourself swimming laps, continuing to use the backstroke or switching to any other stroke you wish. You may feel yourself work up a sweat. Feel your neck stay relaxed as you take regular breaths. When you have swum as many laps as you wish, begin to swim slower and cool down.

Feel how much warmer the water feels now after your more vigorous swimming. Float for a few moments and just soak up the feeling of your body in the water. You are fully supported, luxuriating in the feeling of being completely relaxed. Finally, begin to be aware of the other swimmers.

When you are ready, gently bring your mental movie to an end. See a smile on your face as you finish swimming and get out of the pool. Watch yourself walk confidently to the locker room. Bring your attention back into the room you are lying in. Allow your breathing to continue in a relaxed way for a little while. When you are ready, gently sit up.

Do you feel as though you really had a vigorous swim? Could you feel your body relax and then move through the water? If this was your first attempt at visualization, you may not have been totally absorbed. As with learning any skill, practice will help. This kind of exercise is most effective when you can get as realistic as possible with your images. Trying to see, feel, hear, and touch your surroundings as much as possible will make the scene more real and more effective. Using the same basic technique, you can practice any movement you want, from a dance movement to a tennis stroke. The most important thing is to see yourself clearly in the picture doing exactly what you want to do successfully.

Another way mental imaging works is by creating pictures in your mind that will help you with whatever you're doing. For instance, if you are walking up a hill and feel as though you need a little help, visualize a strong, purposeful wind at your back or a large hand gently supporting you as you go uphill. Sometimes when you are immersed in a strenuous aerobic activity such as running or swimming, an image may pop into your mind uninvited. These images can be simply fun or can be a window inward to help you learn more about yourself. They may not necessarily be positive images, but you can put them to use in a positive way. Once when I was running down a hill an image appeared in my head of a stagecoach with a team of horses running wild and a tiny little me holding the reins and screaming for them to stop. It was as if the image itself was holding me back for fear that I would "run wild." When I manipulated the image, took hold of the reins, and began urging the horses on, my running stride became stronger, and I felt the galloping gait of the horses take me over. Sounds crazy, I know, but it worked, and many people have similar stories to tell.

If you'd like to learn more about imaging and visualization for physical activities, job interviewing, or anything else, there are many books on the subject. Learning to focus your mind is one of the most powerful tools your body has.

Becoming Your Own Coach

Whenever the thought of a winning Olympic athlete comes to mind, you will usually see standing there right next to her a beaming coach. Unfortunately, some athletes report poor relationships with winning-is-the-only-thing coaches who try to shame or guilt-trip them into greater performances. Bad coaching may be worse than none at all. In any event, the ideal coach is the voice of Self-Two. What if we all had such a coach—to teach us the skills we need to play; to see our natural ability and nurture that, not our doubts; to help us try for just a bit more when we think we're too tired and can't; to rejoice with us in our accomplishments; to help us laugh when we begin to take ourselves too seriously. Most of us never had this kind of coaching, but it still can be ours. We can train our own internal coach and then learn to coach ourselves and one another.

Let's start with learning the skills we need to play. Many sports involve throwing a ball. Unless you've specifically been taught, you may use only your arm, and not your whole body, in the throwing motion, in which case someone might say: "You throw like a girl." This phrase is usually used to insult boys, and is based on the idea that males are, and should be, automatically better at sport than females. But there is nothing genetic that makes boys better than girls at throwing; it is a human skill that must be learned in stages. Using only one's arm to throw is a natural stage of development until further training is provided. Many girls do not receive the necessary further training. But it's never too late to try to learn, and you may be able to teach yourself like I did.

I learned to throw a softball, not from our team coach, by the way, but from a suggestion from woman who came regularly to watch our games. I was playing third base, which meant I had to throw from third to first, the longest throw in the infield. After an inning where I'd been short on the throw four times, the woman in the bleachers called me over. "Don't just use your arm and push the ball. Rare back and use your whole body. Watch how some of the others do it and try."

I did. I made a career of going to games and watching others make that throw from third to first. After a good throw I'd close my eyes and get a clear mental picture of how the person's body looked during the throw. Then I'd substitute myself in the picture. Afterwards I'd practice throwing every chance I got. Gradually, after a great deal of mental and physical practice, I began to throw fast, hard, and relatively accurately. I learned that when I "pushed" the ball I bent my arm in front of my shoulder and used only my forearm and wrist for the throw, like a bride tossing her bouquet. No wonder the ball couldn't make it to first! Through visualizing and practice I learned to use my whole body—my arm, shoulder, and back working together so that when I would wind up, my arm would curl behind my shoulder, not in front of it, and end up fully extended in front of me in a full follow-through. I also used my legs, taking a step forward each time I threw and planting my feet for solidity. The throw went to first fueled by my whole body, not just my arm. With the help of my friend in the stands and the skills I learned through sport psychology, I coached myself. I increased my awareness of what I was doing, watched others who knew the skill, planted a vision of them in my mind, and then practiced. And I learned to throw like a third-base player!

I remembered this lesson one day recently when I went for a walk at the beach. A young fellow with a football was trying to entice anyone going by to join him in a game of catch. Footballs are different animals from softballs because they are so much bigger and thus harder to get your hand around, but I'd watched San Francisco Forty-niner quarterback Joe Montana enough to know what a spiral pass was supposed to look like. And I'd learned enough from my bounce-hit tennis days to concentrate on watching the ball as it headed toward me so that I could catch it. Without even really thinking about it I started playing. Catching was no problem. My passes, though, were wobbly at first. But after about four tries, I threw a perfect spiral right to the guy! I could feel my whole body engage in the motion and my arm extend in the follow-through. The ball hit its mark. Thank you, Joe Montana!

I had a great time spontaneously doing something that ten years ago I would never even have tried for fear of embarrassing myself. Because I'd learned to coach myself, I just took a deep breath, applied what I'd learned about throwing, and heard my inner coach say, "Sure you can do it. It'll be fun." And it was. Over the years I've replaced my almost automatic "I can't" or "I won't" with "I'll try." Even though my body told me via aches and pains the next day that it had been quite a while since I'd done any throwing, there was a satisfying little spark of accomplishment that stayed with me and still makes me smile.

You can use similar coaching techniques to help yourself along in any activity. While you're walking, for instance, your coach (who never talks like Self-One) may say, "Remember to breathe, full and relaxed." If you set off to climb to the top of a hill and tire along the way, rather than automatically quitting you might hear your coach saying, "Look around, listen to the birds, feel the ground under your feet, try to exhale every other time your right foot hits the ground." Your Self-One voice might say, "You lazy quitter, get going and no complaining." But Self-Two, your ideal coach, doesn't use negative techniques. She helps you to relax and to develop your body awareness and concentration by turning your attention to your breathing, to specific components of your movement—for example, how the muscles in your thighs are working or the length of your stride. In this way your inner coach helps you go beyond what you thought were your limitations. And when you get to the top of the hill, your coach will be there cheering you on.

Some sports involve more than just changing your attitude and developing your own coaching ability. Some require reflexes you may not have developed while growing up. I was able to learn to throw and catch relatively easily because I'd learned to use my total body and developed hand-eye coordination playing tennis. A friend of mine differentiates between "hand" sports (those requiring balls, bats, rackets, and the like) and "foot" sports (skiing, running, hiking). She sticks with "foot" sports because she doesn't care to take the time to develop the skills for the others. Regardless of what kind of sports you choose, if you give yourself the benefit of the doubt while learning and encourage the development of your internal coach, you are more likely to enjoy yourself. You may want to try simpler or more familiar activities at first and branch out later. For instance, softball requires running around the bases; if you're not able to run now, it's not the sport to start with. But you could still learn to like a game of catch, particularly if you played catch as a child. In any event, positive self-coaching can help you in any activity you choose.

Some of you may be skeptical and feel a bit weird listening to an invisible coaching friend. This is not for everyone, to be sure. But if you hear a strong, critical, judgmental voice in your head, one who only tells you what you're doing wrong rather than encouraging you to learn and try your best, then you should think about replacing that voice and getting a better coach. It's no weirder to listen to a voice that can help you than to listen to that negative voice that can only hurt you. If you're interested, give it a try.

We hope that trying the exercises introduced here will start you on your way to exploring activity with more self-awareness and less self-criticism. There are many more concepts and skills to learn once your curiosity is stimulated. Playing a sport or learning any new physical movement, if done with a focus that includes internal awareness, can be a direct route to learning more about your whole self—body, mind, and emotions. While we have been conditioned to believe that our body stands in our way, often the self-limiting ideas about our potential are the real culprits. World-record-setting marathon swimmer Lynne Cox says that her sport is 10 percent physical and 90 percent mental; many other athletes would no doubt agree. Once you learn the physical basics, training your mind to work for you can become the most important way to stay interested, keep moving, and enjoy yourself. No matter what activity you are trying to learn, nurturing a Self-Two voice may be the best medicine available to begin to heal the damage created by negative body image messages that so many of us have lived with for so long. Besides, it's a lot more fun to play once the crabby judge Self-One is firmly benched.

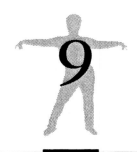

Pitfalls, Detours, Comebacks

How to Keep Yourself Motivated

So you're fired up. Ready to run out the door. What could possibly stop you? The hardest thing is getting your spiffy new shoes laced up, right? Getting out the door regularly is a challenge you're ready for now.

But where does motivation to exercise regularly come from when the initial glow wears off and you become bored or when you experience aches and pains or when you just don't feel like exercising at all? And what if you get up and run out the door right into an injury, which is, unfortunately, all too common for beginning exercisers? And what about all those secret fears that someone will humiliate you by making fun of your big butt? And what if you've already been out there and have quit, for whatever reason, and feel it's just too hard to get started again? That is what this chapter is all about—the common pitfalls, detours, and comebacks that most people experience while integrating exercise into their lives, particularly those fears and misgivings common to larger women.

There are significant barriers to overcome in becoming more active, including the ones discussed earlier, and you may feel that paying attention to others here may actually be counterproductive.

You're raring to go, and we're telling you this feeling can't last forever. Why? Because you are more likely to succeed in the long run if you prepare yourself for the obstacles now. The typical process that people go through—gearing up for aerobics six times a week or walking two hours every day, buying an expensive membership at a health club, taking endless measurements of their bodies and expecting dramatic change, or making a million charts and graphs—*fails*. Two or three weeks after a dive into a regimen like this, most people either burn out or get injured and return to their old, familiar, inactive life-style. The change was too radical, the expectations too unrealistic. It is as if they trained for a sprint when the race was a marathon. Now, to make matters worse, they also have to deal with feelings of being a failure at something they tried so hard to do.

If you sense your "self-improvement" urge being threatened right now—good! It is a short-term motivator with a built-in backfire. Permanent change is most beneficial for both health and self-esteem, and it takes motivation that *lasts*.

For your motivation to exercise to last you need to find the part of you that really enjoys the sheer exuberance of being active. This will take time. You also need to be truthful with yourself about what dampens that spirit so that you can at least try to keep those things away or deal with them realistically when they do occur. Ignoring your feelings of misgiving will not help. It's like saying to yourself, "Well, even if all my other diets failed, this one will surely work," and forging ahead without regard for those nagging feelings of futility. If you have tried a "surefire, quick-start, miracle-cure" exercise program in the past and failed, and who hasn't, you know what we mean. Give yourself a better chance at success this time around.

Fear of Humiliation

There is probably not a fat woman alive who has not experienced a rush of fear while wondering what others will think, do, or say to her when she goes walking or to an exercise or dance class. This fear probably keeps more large women inactive than any other factor, even the fear of injury. It is as if splitting our pants or having someone laugh at us would be more painful than breaking a leg. This is because most of us know how emotionally painful shame and embarrassment are, having experienced them many times before; whereas physical pain may actually seem trivial by comparison, particularly if we have never experienced it. The emotional pain, shame, and humiliation that most of us fat women must endure as a regular, ongoing part of our lives is very real and cannot be ignored or trivialized. Thinner people accuse us of exaggerating, but we are not exaggerating. We can never hope to get beyond this fear, however, unless we face it directly.

What's the most humiliating thing that could happen to you when trying a new activity? Want to hear some real doozies that other women have experienced? One woman tells the story of summoning up her courage to start swimming regularly and going to a local pool. In the locker room, even before she had a chance to get in the pool, an angry woman came up to her, shaking her fist and hissing: "You should be ashamed of yourself. How dare you show yourself in public the way you look. You're disgusting." Talk about dampening enthusiasm! Another woman spoke of attempts to go walking in her neighborhood. Three ten-year-olds kept following her, calling her a fat pig and making oinking noises.

The most amazing part of these stories is not so much that they happened—we know all too well how insensitive people can be—but that the women involved didn't pulverize the perpetrators! Not only are we supposed to endure the most crude and cutting remarks but we're supposed to slink away without committing homicide. It is an unspoken presumption that as fat people we deserve this kind of treatment and will simply have to go on in spite of it. Granted that going to the opposite extreme and advocating violence will not solve anything, but instead of ignoring the feelings of rage that these situations create, you must respond in some way. Even if you cannot summon words to deal with the situation immediately, there is nothing to stop you from fantasizing the worst for those who hurt you when you get home. It not only gives release to your totally justifiable angry feelings but keeps you out of jail.

But fantasizing is not all you can do. There are ways of preparing for these incidents in advance, dealing with them on the spot, and surviving them afterwards. The one thing you must not do is to accept abuse silently and give a home to the feelings of anger, sadness, and shame that fester within and immobilize you.

To arm yourself in advance, try to imagine the worst, most humiliating thing that could happen to you. Once you have confronted that in your mind, you can face comparable real-life scenarios more easily. When you envision the disaster, also try to imagine your responses. You know how you always come up with your best lines after the fact, well this exercise lets you come up with them ahead of the fact. And chances are that if you choose to respond to an insult when it actually happens, the lines you prepared in advance will suit the purpose just fine. The repertoire of "fat lady" insults is amazingly limited and dull. It's easy to be ready for them, but the choice of how to respond is yours. You can be witty, you can terrify someone by hurling abuse in return, you can be dignified and aloof and ignore the creep, or you can tell him or her to go to hell. It's up to you, but whatever you choose to do or not do, be sure to get the incident off your chest after it has occurred. Don't brood over it.

For instance, you can call a friend as soon after an incident as possible and tell her or him every last detail, even the parts that shamed or embarrassed you the most. This is helpful because, among other reasons, if you begin to doubt the legitimacy of being angry, a friend can remind you that you have every right to your anger, sadness, or any other feelings. If you can't reach a friend right away to talk it over with, write it all down on a piece of paper—the incident and all your feelings about it. You may think that "reliving" it will be harder than forgetting it, but this is not so, particularly if the situation hurt you deeply. Reliving it fully on paper or with a friend is the best way to get it out of your system once and for all. Then as soon as possible after reliving it do something good for yourself—treat yourself to a warm bath, a massage, a good movie; buy yourself flowers or play with a child who loves you. Do *not* buy into the idea that anyone has a right to try to shame you, that somehow you "deserved" mistreatment because you are fat. No one ever deserves mistreatment.

It is ironic that while the world screams at fat women to exercise (to lose weight, of course), when we do go out we have to prepare ourselves to deal with insults from all directions. But we must not give up; in fact, the more we are all out there, the more "normal" it will become and the more support we will have for being active. Anyway, having said all this about the cruelty of the world, we have to backtrack and remind you that people can surprise you in nice as well as horrible ways. Strangers often offer smiles of greeting and encouragement, believe it or not. And you can often initiate this response by offering a smile yourself first. But even when crummy incidents do occur, they should not be allowed to deprive us of our right to live with respect in the world. We have a right to take up space, live fully in our bodies and fully in our lives. By dealing with our feelings honestly and supporting one another in this right, we make it easier for ourselves and for those who will follow in our footsteps. If our daughters are going to be able to live active lives, we must blaze a trail for them.

Fear of Injury

Fear of injury ranks right up there as a major barrier to getting started on a more active life. Fear of injury is common for many adults beginning a new activity and can be either realistic or unrealistic. Realistic fear can protect us; it can keep us from setting off on a hike during a blizzard, for example. But unrealistic fear may confine you quite unnecessarily to inactivity. It is up to you to determine which is which and find the level of safety you need to feel confident and avoid injury. One way of doing this is to list all your fears and then analyze them, as suggested in Chapter 2. Once you become more active you may find new fears you didn't think of before you started. You can simply repeat the exercise for any new fears that come up so that they won't stop you.

Analyzing fears also involves asking yourself how you can protect yourself from the injuries you fear. This is particularly important with respect to your heart, which is at risk if proper precautions are not observed during exercise (and before and after as well). One precaution recommended by most exercise advocates to people who have been inactive or who are over thirty-five years of age is to get a complete physical before beginning. While it's hard to disagree with this advice, most people don't follow it. In a practical sense there is very little that a routine physical exam can predict about how well you will do in an exercise program unless a stress electrocardiogram (EKG or ECG) is done as part of the exam, which it usually isn't. The stress EKG is different from the EKG taken at rest, which can only tell you whether your heart has been damaged in the past. A stress EKG records heart activity while you walk on a treadmill, and it is really the only way to find out the true nature of the health of your heart *during exercise,* which is the vital piece of information you need.

Without a stress EKG a general physical exam can give you only minimal information and should not lull you into a false sense of security. If you want a stress EKG, request it. If your doctor doesn't have the equipment in the office, s/he can send you to a special clinic or medical center that does. In some communities the local Y has facilities for doing the stress test. Wherever you go, be sure to get a referral from someone you trust in order to avoid the unsafe testing that some of the more slipshod clinics do. Regardless of whether you get an EKG or not, it is up to you to learn how to take your exercise pulse so you can be sure on a daily basis that you are exercising at a safe heart rate.

Once you take safety precautions for your heart, the next most obvious concern is to prevent injuries to your back, joints, muscles, and tendons. Again, a physical exam is unlikely to give you much useful information to predict how well these parts of your body will do during exercise. It is estimated that 50 percent of Americans experience some difficulty with back problems, so no matter what kind of activity you choose, it's extremely important to learn and use the strengthening exercises for your back and abdominal muscles found in Chapter 4 or in Judy Alter's book, *Surviving Exercise.*

Aside from making sure that you have strong back and abdominal muscles, and enough flexibility to accomplish the movements required for the activities you choose, the keys to preventing injuries to other muscles, joints, and tendons are as follows: not doing too much too soon; warming up and cooling down properly; stretching warmed muscles adequately after exercise; getting qualified instruction; using proper equipment; and learning about your own body. Learning to listen to your body and its feedback mechanisms—how your muscles and joints feel when doing a move, whether you are tensing and holding back—may require lessons and feedback from an instructor in the beginning until you get to know more about how your body is supposed to feel doing certain movements. The stronger and more flexible you become overall, the greater your chances of avoiding injury.

Once you master the basics you can move on to more challenging activities if you wish, but starting out gradually is of utmost importance. Injuries are particularly likely to occur when you abruptly change your routine. For instance, if you usually walk on mostly flat surfaces but one day decide to trek up a steep hill, you may experience pain in your calf muscles or Achilles tendons. Common sense dictates gradual changes in your routine.

Common sense is also helpful when you are trying to figure out why you may be experiencing pain now when you haven't in the past. Perhaps your shoes have worn out and you need a new pair. Or perhaps you need to alter your exercise pattern or location. Let's say you have decided to exercise by walking the two miles to your job every day and taking the bus home, but your regular two-mile route is on a path that, instead of being completely flat and even, slopes downward to one side or the other so that your feet land slightly off balance with each step. Over time you may develop pain in an ankle, knee, or hip from the seemingly slight but nonetheless consistent strain created by walking on an uneven, sloping surface. Instead of giving up, try walking home from work on alternate days. Just balancing the amount of time you walk in each direction might make the difference, or you just may need to find a better route. Don't always jump to the conclusion that you need to stop moving to avoid pain. Sometimes just changing your routine can work the problem out naturally. But anytime you experience sharp, sudden pain it is a clear message to stop and check it out.

Oftentimes our weight is blamed when an injury occurs because fat people are assumed to be clumsy. A thin person can fall off a curb and break her ankle, and no one would assume it happened because of her weight. Let that happen to us and immediately our weight becomes the culprit. But any reading of the sports page will show you how frequently injury sidetracks even elite athletes. It is no embarrassment to be injured, so don't let your feelings get in the way of proper medical treatment if it becomes necessary. Proper treatment is vital for injuries, and don't forget the advice offered earlier to rest, elevate, and ice an injury immediately after it occurs and to avoid localized heat such as from heating pads. Once you take the proper steps initially, time becomes the body's natural healer. If you do become injured, don't be too discouraged—it is a temporary condition. Your body *will* heal, and you will be able to become active again. The most important thing about resuming activity after an injury is to start slowly and pay close attention to any symptoms of strain or reinjury.

Learning the difference between realistic and unrealistic fear is a useful skill in many of life's adventures. Mastering your fear of physical activity spills over to other aspects of your life as well. You can build up your courage muscles, and they will stand you in good stead on the playing field, on the job, and in your personal life. It takes courage to challenge fear and come out the winner. Giving yourself credit for the courage it takes to attempt physical risks is a way to build self-esteem. Attempting physical challenges gives you a practice arena to take reasonable risks and stretch your image of your capabilities. There's nothing quite as empowering as looking back and saying, "I was afraid of that?" and chuckling in amazement at how completely the fear has evaporated.

Guilt for Taking Time for Yourself

Starting an exercise program means taking more time for yourself, making a commitment to your own health and happiness for maybe the first time. It may feel very unfamiliar and may take some getting used to. People in your life may resist your efforts to take time for yourself and try to make you feel guilty for taking time away from them. Children are notorious for this, particularly if you are a working mother, as are spouses/partners, bless their hearts. While in theory they surely want you to be as happy and healthy as you can be, in reality they may have come to rely on you to put their needs before yours. After all, women have been socially trained to do that for millennia, and most of us have internalized that expectation even if others don't impose it on us. A shift to taking more time for yourself and putting your needs first occasionally may be unsettling for a while until you and everyone else gets used to it.

Your loved ones may throw roadblocks in your way just as you run out the door to get to an exercise class or go for a walk. Johnny may pick that exact moment to moan that his teacher says you should help him more with his homework. Or your partner may come home from work down in the dumps and want a sympathetic shoulder to cry on. You have just juggled your entire day to squeeze out an exercise hour for yourself and, *ta-da,* guilt rears its ugly head. Whose needs take priority at that moment?

Our answer is: yours. Firmly tell your child or mate that you love him or her, that you want to talk about their troubles and will be glad to do so just as soon as you get back from your exercise. Then leave.

Yes, the people close to you will probably need to spend some time adjusting to your newfound interest in exercise. They may even belittle your efforts or not take you seriously in a subconscious effort to keep you available to them. Do not expect them to magically transform themselves into self-reliant, super-supportive types overnight, particularly if you have been there for them twenty-four hours a day until now. Your newfound interest may seem threatening, may seem to be pushing them away. In fact, as you become more active and your self-esteem and energy level improve, you will be in better spirits and probably have more energy for them as well as for yourself. In any event, while change can be difficult for everyone at first, don't let your family guilt-trip you out of doing what you need to do to enhance your health and well-being, and to enjoy your life. You will eventually find a way to balance your needs with theirs.

Guilt, like dieting, helps no one. It is just one more way to feel worthless, and who needs it! This is not to say you won't feel it, but you can make a conscious choice not to act on it. By sticking to your commitment to yourself you enable the people in your life to become more respectful of the needs of others. In the long run they may thank you. But for now don't hold your breath. Write the word GUILT on a piece of paper, burn it, and get on with it.

Living with Aches and Pains

If you have been completely sedentary up until now, you can expect some minor muscle aches and pains as your body adjusts to its newfound movement adventures. Discovering your hidden urge to move may mean learning ways to soothe your body while these urges are being uncovered. The most helpful treatment for the almost inevitable minor muscle aches and pains in the beginning and even well in to an active life is a warm bath or Jacuzzi right after exercising. A warm shower can feel great, too, but your body may really crave soaking up heat for several minutes. This is why Jacuzzis, saunas, and steam rooms are so popular in health clubs.

If you are stiff after your first exercise outing, give your body a day to rest a bit. When you start up your exercise program again, you may still feel a bit stiff and sore even after a day's rest, so just go at a slower pace. Letting your muscles be active again will help any stiffness subside. Slow, gentle stretching can also help. Eventually, as your body gets more used to movement, you will not be bothered by aches and pains as much. Some doctors recommend aspirin for minor aches and pains caused by exercising. You be the judge of how you want to care for yourself.

For some people, living with physical pain is a daily reality although not resulting from a new level of activity. Some large women have back injuries, arthritis, or other painful conditions and may be limited in what they can do as a result of pain. If this is your situation, probably the best solution will be exercising in a warm pool, either walking or swimming, and then doing gentle stretches. A limited range of motion often can be expanded with gentle exercise. But to be on the safe side you may need to find a physical therapist who will not simply blame your problem on your weight and tell you to go on a diet but will work with you to design an exercise routine that will allow you to be as active as you can be.

Another kind of pain that can come up during exercise is emotional pain, and it can come as a complete surprise. At a Radiance Retreat, the We Dance class was a big hit, with most of the women joining in the fun. A few women left in the middle of the class, though. Later they revealed how much pain they experienced when dancing. They had never been asked to dance or go to proms as teenagers, had always been told they were too fat to be attractive, and had been excluded from dancing. As adults, then, when their bodies started moving in the dance, this long-buried pain was triggered along with the desire to be included.

Fortunately there were other women at the retreat with whom

they could cry and share their feelings instead of suppressing them, which would have compounded both the pain and the isolation. Do not be surprised if you, too, experience strong emotion as a result of being more active. Suppressed emotional pain seems like a given for many fat women. Whether it is related to incidents in childhood or more recent times, it seems to lie close to the surface where it can be easily triggered into consciousness. Since physical activity often does seem to act as that trigger, remember the sturdy Girl Scout motto and *be prepared* for the pain. That does not mean fearing or avoiding it. You might even welcome it for the opportunity it gives you to explore it and come to terms with it. Getting support for dealing with your pain directly is the best thing you can do for yourself. If you simply suppress it again, you can indeed shove it back below the surface of consciousness, but then it will always be there, awaiting the signal—a dance class, a cruel remark, whatever—to surface again. So reach out to people. You'll be surprised how many of them have experienced the same feelings and have gotten past them.

Setting Aside Cultural Expectations

We have talked about some of the cultural barriers that need to be overcome en route to becoming more active. Strongest among these perhaps is the current cultural imperative to "lose weight and get in shape" that comes at us from every direction—doctors, family, friends, Madison Avenue, Jane Fonda, Richard Simmons, and other total strangers. The current cultural fascination with fitness may act as a barrier rather than an incentive because to "comply" by becoming more active may seem to be caving in to the assessment that you are not okay just the way you are. Women who choose not to be constantly vigilant about their appearance—those who are not obsessed with the latest fashions, makeup, and nail polish colors—may be accused of not being "feminine enough." It seems wise at this point to examine the influence of cultural expectations on motivation.

As children we had to obey whether we wanted to or not. As adolescents we usually rebelled against doing precisely those things we were told to do. In both cases we let what others wanted determine our behavior—first by complying, later by resisting. As adults we have the capacity to assert an agenda of our own, independent of others' desires for us. But it takes some real strength in your own goals to be able to do what the world wants you to but for your own reasons. This means that if your family or your doctor or your boss is on your back to "get in shape," you can expect to find a mule kick inside you just waiting to happen.

You need to know and *believe* two things. First, what "they" want you to do is not necessarily what you have to want for yourself. Girls are socialized to be very sensitive to other people's wishes and to make those agendas their own in order to please. Conversely, teenagers are very sensitive to other people's wishes and reject them on that basis in order to feel independent. As an adult, you have a *choice*. Be clear about which of the reasons for exercising are yours and which are other people's. They can be the same or different; what matters is that your reasons, your motivation to exercise is yours, not theirs.

Second, you have a *right* to the pleasure of movement. You may be tired of hearing us say this, but it is so easy to forget! We have been deprived of opportunities to be active both as females and as fat people. The fitness culture offers us a mockery of truly satisfying activity—the saccharine substitute for the honey of exuberant, sweaty, playful dance and sport. Physical activity motivated by "self-improvement" is a house of cards. Build your foundation on the innate desire of your body to *move*. What kind, with whom, where, when and, most important, why are decisions that only you can make, and you need no one's approval for your choices.

Looking for Inspiration?

Now that we have covered some of the common concerns or pitfalls you could encounter when becoming more active, it's a good idea to remember that all of the angst and disruption becoming more active may entail is definitely worth it. Becoming more active can change your life for the better. This may seem to contradict our suggestion not to focus on "self-improvement" as a motivator. It is not. You are a fine person now, in need of no "self-improvement" to value yourself, but that is not to say your life cannot be more enjoyable than it is. Becoming more active may simply increase your options for enjoyable activities. It may inspire you to go beyond anything you might imagine for yourself right now. And most of us can use a good jolt of inspiration on occasion.

When we decided to write this book several women contacted us, wanting to contribute their stories about being fat and fit, and how they got that way. In addition to all of the women in the Bay

Area we talked with, one of the people we heard from was Lee Eastman who lives in Cornelius, Oregon. Her words tell her story best.

I'm glad to know I'm not the only one who thinks fat does not rule out being fit or participating in a chosen sport. I encourage anyone I talk to to find their activity and go for it. Who cares what "they" say as long as we're having fun and feeling good?

I'm one of those people who has been fat all her life. Right now I'm thirty-one years old, stand five feet nine and a half inches tall, weigh 305, wear a size 50 blouse and 44–46 slacks. When I was growing up my mom tried to make being fat all right by telling me I was active and solid, not flabby. But I was still teased at school and felt self-conscious, so I started dieting. Would you believe my first diet was at age eleven? I shudder to think what it did to my body then. My last diet at age twenty almost killed me. But thankfully it was my last one. I told myself I had given it my best shot, and I was doomed to be fat. I stopped weighing myself and stopped denying myself all the foods I liked. Of course the pounds came back and brought some friends. But I bought larger clothes and set out to learn to like myself as I was. I succeeded. I do like myself, and that is what started me exercising. I like myself enough to want to do good things for me, and this is just one of them.

I first went to a local exercise studio to a class for the Overweight and Out of Shape, knowing I would never be a size 3. I decided to be me, no matter what a skinny instructor said (I knew she would be skinny and unsympathetic, out to rid the world of us fatties), and was really surprised when the instructors didn't put us down or try to put us on diets. They encouraged us, had us do what we could, and shared our successes with the class. They were willing to work with us, modifying the exercises and routines as needed. And so I became one of their biggest supporters and went to the class for over a year.

While those of us in the class liked the instructors, we thought the class would be perfect if we could get a large-sized instructor. When we brought it up to the current instructors they agreed, and the next thing I knew I was being trained to teach the class and now am certified as a dance-exercise instructor! I changed the name of the class to Large and Lovely because I objected to being called overweight and out of shape. Now my classes are well received, and people seem to enjoy seeing someone who looks just like them teaching them about exercise.

On a personal level, the changes in my life are everywhere! One of the first things I noticed was that I slept better, had more energy, and didn't feel as though I would fall asleep the moment I sat down after work as had often happened before. I now *want* to walk places and take the stairs, and will take a parking space out in the boonies rather than park closer. I feel capable, more self-confident and assured, and find myself doing things that in the past I would have waited for my husband to do for me.

My body has changed considerably too. I am two dress sizes smaller and can now go into a store and buy things off the rack rather than having to rely only on catalogues that carry my size. I have fantastic calves now and look great in a skirt! When I started exercising I was so swaybacked I couldn't press my lower back to the floor. Now I can get my back down there, and I stand a quarter inch taller than I did. I am more aware of my body and what it is telling me, and I have finally discovered the difference between stomach hunger and mouth hunger that all those dieting demons always talk about.

Having made a commitment to fitness, I found myself making other changes in my life as well. Diet is a four-letter word for me. If I think of dieting, my body turns mule and digs in its feet. Even before I start I feel deprived. But I have made changes in my eating. My food choices are more healthy. I've cut down salt and fat and have increased my fiber intake and am aware of my calcium levels. It hit me one day that I was working so hard to get my body healthy I should pay attention to its nutritional needs as well. But I didn't make all these changes overnight. I took it one day at a time. Mind you, I don't turn down ice cream when it's offered or munch celery sticks when my body is screaming for a Hershey bar with almonds! But my cravings have changed, and I no longer view certain foods as bad or good. A big green salad is as much a treat for me now as chocolate cake or a bag of potato chips.

I am also more willing to take risks now. I go to these workshops for aerobics instructors and know I will be the biggest person there. But I don't let it stop me. I say to myself, "If people can't accept me as I am, it's their problem, not mine," and I believe it. I am an instructor, too, and my classes deserve the best teacher they can get. I have as much right and reason to be there as the rest of them. One thing I am adamant about in my class, though, is not emphasizing weight loss. If I had my way, all bathroom scales would be destroyed! I encourage my class to judge their progress on how they feel rather than any changes in numbers on that monster in the bathroom. I see myself getting into my leotard and heading out for the gym when I am eighty because fitness for me is a lifetime commitment. I am participating in more fun runs (I walk them so they will stay fun for me) and am taking care of my body because I now realize how long I want it to last. And I feel as if I could burst with all the positive things I want to share with other large women. Most important is that we can be fit and fat and *healthy* and all without killing ourselves with one diet after another!

The Magic Word: Motivation

What is it that can keep us from doing what is clearly in our best interest? What is it that could stimulate us just right so we could make a commitment to ourselves, smile, and go out and join the Lee Eastmans of the world and have fun? Where's that magic pill called motivation, and where can I sign up for regular doses? you might be thinking.

Well, as you already know, there is no magic pill called "motivation." We hope we have dispelled the notion of exercise as a cure-all for all your problems—even in the midst of sharing stories from women like Lee whose lives have changed dramatically—because viewing any one thing as a cure-all dooms you to failure. Sweaty fun is just that—not a cure-all but well worth the effort. There is no single idea or inspiration that motivates everyone into action. What motivates individuals is as varied as we all are. There do seem to be common elements, however, and we'll share some of them with you because what has worked for us and for some of the other women we know may work for you too.

Sometimes what entices people is the pure joy of the idea of being in great shape and the challenge and commitment to yourself it would take to get there. Without the dual forces of challenge and commitment it is difficult to stay with a long-term goal, particularly when you do not notice positive changes right away. Initially you may notice only aches and pains. To stick with it means letting go of our red-blooded American tendency to want instant gratification. To nurture a vision of ourselves as strong, full of energy, flexible, more in tune with the world and with ourselves is valuable as a way of sustaining ourselves when in doubt, but it may be a pure act of faith if you haven't had the experience firsthand of being in great shape. It therefore does not replace the need to enjoy yourself as much as possible in the present.

So once again it comes to choosing activities that you think you will like and sticking with them long enough to see if you do. Going to a dance class or for a walk once and deciding it is not for you is not really giving yourself a fair chance. Very soon, perhaps in six weeks or so, you will begin to see positive change—in your energy level, flexibility, strength, attitude—and it will add to your incentive. It's also extremely helpful to have a partner to exercise with during the first six weeks. It can have the effect of doubling your motivation because while you might let yourself slide, if someone else is counting on you there's a greater incentive to follow through on your original commitment. But probably the most important part of motivating yourself in the beginning is finding something in the present moment of the activity to give you pleasure while you remain committed to longer term goals.

We've made a list of what women have told us they use for motivation. The "I" is not the same person in these examples, nor does the same reason necessarily work every day. It's good to know that lots of different reasons work at different times to get you going.

- Some days it's knowing I'm going to see something beautiful—a sunset, the ocean, a stream, a flower in bloom, trees turning their fall colors. The great outdoors can get me out there like nothing else. I love the silence, the smells, the beauty, the grounded feeling I get when I'm outside. It helps me put things into perspective, particularly when I get hung up in petty problems. I think of myself as just another speck in the universe, and there's something really peaceful in that.

- I know I'll see people I like and have a good time with when I go to my dance class. We talk over our lives or just schmooz, take time to laugh and get silly, or ask for serious support. Sometimes just being with them is what matters, particularly if I'm feeling lonely, out of sorts, or alienated. Other times, if I'm feeling great and want to share that with others and have fun, that's possible too. And believe me, they are an inspiring bunch to be with!

- I love the physical release, the sweating, the trying for more, the being totally satisfied that I have moved every muscle and awakened all my blood cells. I feel alive! I've stressed my body, made my heart beat, had my chest open up with deep breaths. I got rid of the stiffness that comes from too much slouching over a computer and feel my whole self loosen up and get more flexible. When my body loosens up, so does my mind and my mood.

- My life gets so hectic that I just need solitude and go for walks alone. It's a time to be quiet, with no phones ringing, no demands, just time for me. If I need to think about a problem, I can sift and sort it, look at it from a different angle, let another voice (not my usual sitting-down-stuck voice) give it a go. "Don't trust a thought that comes to you when you're sitting down" urges me to move, think on my feet, and often gets me unstuck. Sometimes I get a flash of inspiration and the problem is solved. Or I may just see it differently. Most of the time, though, I try not to think about problems and just appreciate letting all problems drift away for at least the time of my walk. There seems to be plenty of time to work on problems during the rest of my life so I can just enjoy the peace of my walking time.

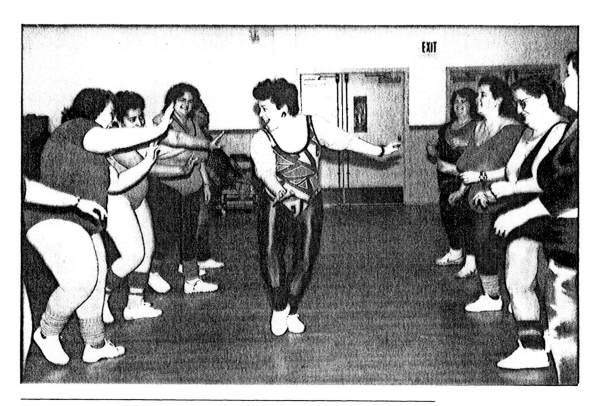

Egging on and hamming it up at We Dance.

- I may need to cry about something, get rid of whatever it is that's bogging me down. Some hidden melancholy. Sometimes it helps just to move my molecules around some, shake myself up, shake loose the veneer of control, and let go. Sometimes I don't even know I'm sad or upset until I've been moving for a while, and then slowly the tears may come. I'm no longer afraid to let the tears happen. Washing away any sad feelings when I'm moving is a low-risk, low-cost kind of therapy.

- Sometimes I just know I will feel better when I get through. That's all. I'll feel as though I've accomplished something, particularly when I'm tired and out of sorts. After a workday, when I feel as if all I want to do is collapse, I say to myself: "Not on my time—on my time I want to be awake." Why give alert, energetic time only to others, to a job, even if it's a job I love? I heard someone say that "a good job can't love you back, so why give it all your time and energy?" It struck home. Sometimes I just have to get back to me, and sweating and getting physical gets me back to me, gets me back to what I want for myself.

♦ I guess I'm just ornery and want to become more fit and healthy because other people think I can't. They are amazed that I'm still walking my four days a week more than a year after I started. They're sitting there saying what an inspiration I am. It is weird and nice at the same time to be an inspiration. I guess it's just the chip on my shoulder that says, "Oh, yeah," and gets me out there to prove to them and to myself that I can go beyond limited stereotypes and expectations—both theirs and mine. I guess it's the one time the chip on my shoulder helps me!

♦ Sometimes I just need a safe way to blow off steam. To pound softballs into the outfield. To pound tennis balls into a backboard and see my boss's sickening smile on each ball. When I'm angry it helps just to smash things for a bit, and then I feel better. I can get back to a more even keel and not be so upset.

♦ I began to swim regularly out of desperation. I just didn't know what else to do. I'd tried everything else to treat back pain from an injury that was making me more and more immobile every day. I was terrified of spending the rest of my life flat on my back. A large woman friend of mine changed her mobility completely through swimming, and I thought that if it worked for her maybe it could work for me. It did. Now whenever I doubt whether I have the energy to go swimming I remember how immobile I was before and just go. It's not a question of asking myself whether I want to swim today or not. I just do it, and once I'm in the water it's always worth it because I can move so freely.

♦ I try to go to the fat women's swim every week. I look forward so much to the one time during the week that I can feel completely safe, when I can count on not being harassed or even the tiniest bit insulted about my weight. "They" say it isn't enough to exercise only once a week, that it doesn't do any good. Well "they" haven't been to the swim. It has changed my life. I go every week not even so much for the exercise, although that makes my body feel good, but for the good feelings I leave with in my heart.

♦ I just love the physical feeling that comes from a perfect tennis shot. I just want to feel that place of no thinking, just being, just moving, just doing it. Doing my best because I'm not trying. That's the most fun for me. It keeps me coming back, putting up with all my lousy shots for the feel of that one perfect one. It's great when it happens. Peaceful and exhilarating at the same time.

♦ I like the whole ritual of putting on my sweats and shoes, knowing that the time ahead is just for me. I know after putting in a hard workday that finally it's playtime. And almost every time

I'm out walking I remember the feelings I had crossing the finish line of my first race. I can call up that memory in a second and experience again the joy of being so satisfied and happy. Sure there are times when I wish I could still run, but then I think about all the years before when I just lay around and didn't do anything at all. I may not be going as fast or as far now as I used to, but I'm still going and that's enough. And remembering my "moment of glory" still keeps me walking day after day.

♦ Sometimes I need to not exercise. To say the hell with it for today and lay on the couch. I may feel irritable and out of sorts, or I just may want to lay low. So I give myself permission to be inactive. It keeps me from getting too rigid and compulsive about exercise. But I can't not go for too many days in a row because the longer I'm away from it, the harder it is to get up from a sitting position. It's not impossible, I know, it's just harder. That's why I want to keep going once I start. But sometimes I just can't, and that's okay now. I don't have to be a "perfect exerciser" to enjoy myself.

♦ For me, exercising is not a decision I make every day. I made one decision—to get up in the morning, every morning, in time to walk to work. So I just do it. It's not based on whether I feel like it or not because if I take any time to think about it, I may not do it. It's the commitment to myself over the long haul that silences all those little voices of nagging doubt that could get me off my course if I let them in. I just get up and get out the door before all the little voices are even awake.

♦ I like all the new sports I've learned in the past three years. I can't even remember what I did to keep busy before because now there are just not enough hours in the week to do all the things I like to do. I started out with aerobics because I love music. Now I swim and am getting ready to start a karate class, and on weekends I try to find new places to hike to so I can feel like an explorer. And all because I got tired of huffing and puffing every time I tried to walk up stairs!

♦ Now that I know what it feels like to be in good shape, I want to stay that way. I have lots of energy, and it's easier to do more and enjoy more. Once I got back into totally vegging out for a few months, and it just felt very, very different. It seems to take so long to get going, but if you quit being active, in a flash you're practically back where you started. I heard you lose 50 percent of your fitness level in two weeks by not staying active. I can't let my wanting to veg get in the way of my bigger want—to feel good.

From the comments included here you can see that there are a variety of feelings and ideas which can provide the motivation to become more active, even on those days when maybe your first choice is to let it slide. Until you uncover more and more of your hidden desire to move and you find ways to express that desire in whatever activities you choose, the process of developing interest in exercise may be slow. No problem. It is the slow, gradual change in your overall activity pattern that will be the most lasting. If you can retain your spirit of adventure and play, all the better. If you are fueled by curiosity about what and how much you can do without getting caught up in comparing yourself to others, your main goal will be self-discovery, not self-improvement. It is vital to make this switch in attitude in order to give you a better shot at lasting enjoyment in exercise and movement.

On the Comeback Trail

Fitness, like life, is a series of ongoing changes—maybe even an ongoing series of comebacks—and you cannot assume that once you get into shape you will always stay that way. You may, but then again you may not. So there's no point in putting off the good things in life until you get there, making "in shape" the magical destination weight loss used to be: "When I get 'there' then I'll be happy and treat myself right." "When I get 'there' I'll buy myself some great new clothes that fit." Waiting until you get in shape to treat yourself well will not help you get into shape in the first place, so you might as well just treat yourself well from the beginning.

There's no denying that fitness is a worthwhile destination, albeit something short of magical, and it's true that knowing what being in good shape feels like is motivation for making a comeback and doing it again. In fact, it feels much worse *not* to be in great shape when you know the difference. It's sort of like being depressed all your life, then getting some help or making some positive changes until one day you wake up and say, "I'm happy!" and realize it is a feeling totally different from any you've had before. It's easy to forget what happiness feels like when you've been depressed for a long time, but after not being depressed for a while you realize that being happy is better. Happiness may even be a little threatening because it is unfamiliar, but most of us would surely rather be happy than depressed if given the choice. The problem is that it doesn't feel like a choice. To realize we *do* have the power to make changes that will help us feel better can be motivation in itself. Seeing ourselves make a comeback reinforces the idea that we can do it again and again. It can keep us going in the face of very slow progress. And every time we make a positive change our sense of personal power grows even stronger. It becomes a cycle of strength that perpetuates itself.

The most important reason to become more physically active is to please yourself. To give yourself more ways to enjoy your life. To affirm your right to all of the pleasures life has to offer. To be strengthened by your experience and know you can always make a comeback in fitness or in other areas of your life because you have your experience to back you up.

Physical accomplishments are hard to deny. If you start out by swimming half a lap and eventually swim a mile, you can't deny your progress. If your resting pulse goes from eighty to seventy in the space of a year or if your blood pressure has been high and it comes down, this is tangible evidence that your body is changing, becoming more healthy as a result of your exercise choices. We have been geared to measure our success by the scale for so long that to shift our perspective to other numbers that may change—decreases in blood pressure or pulse, increases in number of laughs per day—may be hard to accept at first. It may be difficult to give these new measurements as much value as you have always given your weight. But making this shift is a goal you can work toward, knowing ahead of time that you are likely to succeed.

Recess, Remember?

Even on the days when we are inspired to dance or run or play, there is a slug inside us yearning to be free. It is the slug that needs motivation. The slug, which lives in people of all sizes, just wants to relax and lay on the couch. Nothing violent or anything. Just a simple veg, comforting and familiar. Being a slug is not a criminal act, it is only being a slug, and there are plenty of happy slugs in the world. But for most of us, when we act like slugs we end up feeling slug-ish—stiff, bored, antsy but exhausted. You have to figure out, therefore, how to entice the slug into action even when it may not be her first choice.

It's a well-known scientific fact that even slugs love recess. The little buggers just love the chance to squeal with laughter. So when all else fails to get you going, just try to coax that slug into action by playing some of your favorite childhood games—those old four-square games can still work magic—or even find some kids to play with you. They can help you remember why recess was so enjoyable.

If recess was full of ridicule and teasing when you were a child, trust that it will be better now as an adult. Trust that you can cultivate a more playful attitude over time, that you will come to love it, that it could introduce you to a self you haven't even met yet. A more playful you can take your slug side on adventures you once thought beyond your abilities. Once you get used to adventuring you'll be amazed at what a difference it can make. Many of us have been deprived of experiencing our bodies in motion, and it's high time we asserted our right to play. Strengthen your comeback attitude with hearty doses of laughter—it will help keep your tendencies toward self-improvement in check. It's hard to feel you're working on self-improvement when you're giggling.

Whenever you feel the tendency to whip out the old impossible goals, charts, graphs, and measuring tape, remember the words of the sage: "Life is what happens to you while you're busy making other plans." Plan to enjoy your life right now because you deserve it. Remember that you are your own most powerful resource. Believing the best about yourself today can heal past wounds. Let all of us encourage our daughters and one another to run and dance and play—not just because it helps us all grow healthy and strong but because movement is one of life's simple pleasures and is fun.

We hope you will join in the adventure that a more active life can bring. Listen, that sounds like the recess bell now. . . . Come out, come out, wherever you are. It's time to play!

Annotated Bibliography

General Topic Books with Chapters on Fat Fitness

Boston Women's Health Collective, *The NEW Our Bodies, Ourselves* (New York: Simon and Schuster, 1984). Among the wealth of information presented here is a substantial chapter on women and exercise, with specific sections addressed to disabled women, older women, and fat women. The short series of suggestions for fat women was written by a fat activist and is oriented toward giving readers permission to have fun moving and to let them know they have a right to be physically active in spite of our culture. It stops short of presenting a specific movement program and is necessarily brief.

Jean du Coffe and Sherry Suib Cohen, *Making It Big* (New York: Simon and Schuster, 1980). This book on living fully for large women has a chapter devoted to exercise. The authors present general concerns for larger women as well as a specific calisthenics program designed by Jamie Bourne. It is exciting to see large models demonstrating the exercises, but many of the calisthenics are hazardous for larger bodies, straining joints and emphasizing end-point positions rather than movement directions. The class's instructor informs us that the exercise program has since been updated. Another significant drawback is the program's lack of aerobics.

Nancy Roberts, *Breaking All the Rules* (New York: Penguin Books, 1985). One of the most dynamic and articulate spokeswomen for size acceptance has written a book that covers a tremendous amount of territory, including exercise. This book is packed with inspiration and information, although it doesn't give a specific exercise program.

Fitness for Larger Women

Ann Smith, *The Gifted Figure: Proportioning Exercises for Large Women* (Santa Barbara: Capra Press, 1984). This book incorporates many positive features: stretches tailored for bigger bodies, large model photos, and an emphasis on pleasure and body fitness rather than weight loss. But there are substantial flaws as well. The movements are slow and graceful, inspired by dance and yoga, and are not calculated to build strength or cardiovascular fitness. Some stretches are hazardous, and the author's contention that stretching alone can reapportion fat deposits is debatable. Large women looking for a gentle program of stretching exercises to supplement another program could use many of the movements in this book after learning which are safe from Judy Alter's *Surviving Exercise*.

Bonnie D. Kingsbury, *Full Figure Fitness* (Champaign, Illinois: Life Enhancement Publications, 1988). This book can be used by either the individual exerciser or the instructor looking for helpful ideas on teaching an exercise program for large people. The photos picture large-size models and the text covers the basic concerns of starting a class. The tone of the book is somewhat ambivalent: there are ground-breaking ideas here along with some more conservative stands on obesity and health.

Generic Fitness and Exercise

Judy Alter, *Surviving Exercise* (1983) and *Stretch and Strengthen* (1986), (Boston: Houghton Mifflin Company). The safest and most accessible program for able-bodied people of any size, presenting important information on exercises to perform and exercises to avoid. Although Alter uses slender-bodied line-drawings to demonstrate exercises and makes no mention of specific modifications for fat bodies, her books are quite useful.

Covert Bailey, *Fit or Fat?* (Boston: Houghton Mifflin Company, 1977). The problem with this book is inherent in the title—the assumption that one can be fit *or* fat but not both. Bailey argues that people are fat not because of overeating but because of aerobic inactivity, and he educates readers on the subject of aerobics. While fat people usually do lose some fat by doing aerobic activity, there will be many who remain "overweight" by society's standards, and Bailey's abhorrence of fat compromises the important information he presents. There is as well a lack of information on the particular problems (and how to avoid them) of heavier bodies doing aerobics.

Peter and Lorna Francis, Ph.D.'s, *If It Hurts, Don't Do It* (Rocklin, California: Prima Publishing, 1988). This wonderful little book makes it easy to tailor an exercise program to your body and your lifestyle. The book diagrams common postural misalignments and describes the various stretching and strengthening exercises which can help correct them and gives sound advice on creating an aerobic program of activity for yourself. While they do not specifically address the issue of fatness and fitness, they challenge common misconceptions about weight loss and exercise.

James Garrick, M.D., and Peter Radetsky, *Peak Condition* (New York: Crown Publishers, 1986). A comprehensive and easy-to-understand book on how to prevent, treat, and rehabilitate sports injuries, including aerobic dance injuries. While the authors do not identify issues of particular interest to heavier people, the book's information is very useful.

John Krausz and Vera van der Reis Kraus, *The Bicycling Book* (New York: Dial Press). An amazing encyclopedia of bicycling for transportation, recreation, and sport. The editors present hundreds of articles by teachers, coaches, doctors, engineers, racers, and recreational cyclists on everything from how to buy your first bike to how to train for the most challenging outings.

Charles T. Kuntzleman, *The Complete Book of Walking* (New York: Pocket Books, 1979). While unfortunately emphasizing weight loss as an expected outcome of walking, there is still plenty of sound information to make this well worth the price of $2.95. It offers tips on setting up a training routine, coping with pain, walking in all kinds of weather, and sustaining your enthusiasm.

Joan Ullyot, M.D., *Women's Running* (Mountain View: (California) World Publications, 1976). This is a basic book for beginning runners. If you read around Ullyot's fat phobia, rampant in this and subsequent books and articles, you can glean useful information on getting started and avoiding injuries.

Women in Sport

Arlene Blum, *Annapurna: A Woman's Place* (San Francisco: Sierra Club Books, 1980). The inspiring, exciting account of the first all-women's ascent of a Himalayan mountain. Pertinent for anyone who doubts the ability of women to achieve greatness.

Mary Boutilier and Lucinda San Giovanni, *The Sporting Woman* (Champaign, Illinois: Human Kinetics Publishers, 1983). An inspiring compilation of research on women in sport with an insightful analysis of the barriers to full participation. Includes historical, social, political, psychological, and educational information vital for individuals who wish to empower women through sport. A must for physical education and fitness instructors.

Janice Kaplan, *Women and Sports* (New York: Avon Books, 1979). A rather breezy account of the changes in attitudes and opportunities for women athletes that occurred in the mid to late 1970s. Useful in ridding us of the idea that sports are inappropriate for women and girls, with a particularly interesting discussion of feminism and femininity as it relates to female athletes. Watch out for the standard fat-phobic views.

Stephanie L. Twin, *Out of the Bleachers* (New York: The Feminist Press, 1979). A compilation of writings on various aspects of women in sport, from historical and political perspectives to first-person accounts of women athletes. An inspiration for budding athletes or curious women's history buffs.

Sports Psychology and Alternate
Views of Sport

Timothy Gallwey, *The Inner Game of Tennis* (New York: Random House, 1974). A Zen approach to sport, emphasizing practical ways to heighten awareness and concentration skills. The first and perhaps best of three books written on this approach for different sports, it presents a refreshing plan for getting rid of self-criticizing inner voices that undermine our efforts in sport and in life.

Dorothy V. Harris, Ph.D., and Bette L. Harris, Ed.D., *Sports Psychology: Mental Skills for Physical People* (New York: Leisure Press, 1984). Nuts-and-bolts philosophy and exercises in relaxation and visualization to improve physical performance, particularly during competition. Useful for people who are more seriously interested in developing these skills for participation in their sport.

George Leonard, *The Ultimate Athlete* (New York: Avon Books, 1974). A "revisioning" of sports, physical education, and the body, with an emphasis on creating attitudes and situations that will make sports more available to anyone who wishes to try. Utilizing the philosophy of Akido to maximize the body's energy, Leonard aims to integrate mind, body, and spirit. Incorporates much of the New Games philosophy and offers a perspective different from the competitive Western sports model.

Peter Nabokov, *Indian Running* (Santa Barbara: Capra Press, 1981). A historical account of running in early Indian communities, combined with photos and first-person accounts of the 1980 Tricentennial run commemorating the All-Pueblo Revolt of 1680. Insights into Native American culture reveal an interesting contrast to the macho, competitive attitude of white culture.

Sociological Treatments of Body Size

Kim Chernin, *The Obsession: Reflections on the Tyranny of Slenderness* (New York: Harper and Row, 1981). A fascinating treatise on our culture's obsession with slenderness. The author explores more issues of body size in general than fat people's concerns in particular.

Marcia Millman, *Such a Pretty Face* (New York: Norton, 1980). An excellent sociological study of being fat in America, looking closely at the National Association to Aid Fat Americans, Overeaters Anonymous, and a summer weight-loss camp for teens. The author raises provocative issues about the experience of fat people by using short interview excerpts and observation.

Lisa Schoenfielder and Barb Wieser, eds., *Shadow on a Tightrope* (Iowa City: Aunt Lute, 1983). Writings on fat women's lives, including an excellent thirteen-page section on "the struggle of fat women to be outside, to exercise, to participate in sports." This section covers the experiences of four fat women in swimming, dance, softball, and karate. An important and timely anthology.

Hillel Schwartz, *Never Satisfied: A Cultural History of Diets and Fantasies and Fat* (New York: Free Press, 1986). This book puts the current dieting frenzy in perspective by tracing its historical roots. Very useful for looking critically at what often seems like our "inevitable" or "natural" cultural assumption that everyone should look like Twiggy.

Roberta Pollack Seid, *Never Too Thin: Why Women are at War with Their Bodies* (New Jersey: Prentice Hall, 1989). Seid is a historian and brings both depth and perspective to her discourse on how our society came to the conclusion that thinness should be craved over all else. Extensively referenced.

Body Awareness

Rita Freedman, Ph.D., *Bodylove: Learning to Like Our Looks and Ourselves* (New York: Harper and Row, 1989). A practical guide to changing feelings of body loathing to those of body love, stressing movement as one key tool. A wealth of warmth, wisdom, and inspiring information for any woman at odds with her body.

Marcia Germaine Hutchinson, Ed.D., *Transforming Body Image: Learning to Love the Body You Have* (Trumansburg, New York: Crossing Press, 1985). A more psychologically oriented self-help book presenting a series of visualization exercises designed to help women bring unconscious attitudes to the surface to be worked through. Very comprehensive and interesting. Probably most useful when done with a partner or a group of similarly interested people.

Anne Kent Rush, *Getting Clear: Body Work for Women* (New York: Random House, 1973). One of the best self-help books to come out in the early days of women's health writing. Explores specific ways to accept our bodies, including exercises in breathing, relaxation, and centering. A wealth of insights on how to heighten body awareness and overcome negative body image, presented in a down-to-earth tone with lots of pictures and diagrams. Since it is out of print, check your used-book stores or library.

Advice on Eating and Dieting Disorders

William Bennett, M.D., and Joel Gurin, *Dieters' Dilemma* (New York: Basic Books, 1982). A well-documented account of the pitfalls of dieting as a means of weight loss. Bennett and Gurin assemble the latest medical research to test the hypothesis of "setpoint," that is, the body's investment in maintaining a certain amount of fat in the face of fluctuations in caloric intake. They argue that aerobic exercise is one of the few ways to moderately lower the setpoint setting.

Jane Brody, *Jane Brody's Nutrition Book: A Lifetime Guide to*

Good Eating for Better Health and Weight Control (New York: Bantam Books, 1982). Packed with good common sense about nutrition. Although the book's subtitle refers to weight control, Brody has since written excellent articles on the more recent research on set-point and the hazards of dieting. A very comprehensive book on nutritional facts and practical ways to eat more healthily.

Jane Hirschmann and Carol Munter, *Overcoming Overeating* (New York: Addison-Wesley, 1988). When compulsive dieting has left a legacy of compulsive eating, this book can help you "live free in a world of food." One of the best aspects of this book is a question-and-answer section on the nuts-and-bolts of eating normally.

Jane Hirschmann and Lela Zaphiropoulos, *Are You Hungry? A Completely New Approach to Raising Children Free of Food and Weight Problems* (New York: New American Library, 1987). A common-sense guide to helping your children eat normally in a world that creates dieters out of fourth-graders. Excellent advice to genetically heavier kids and their families about how to take the focus off of weight and instead enhance self-esteem.

Susan Kano, *Making Peace with Food (Revised Edition)* (New York: Harper and Row, 1989). This workbook is full of excellent exercises to understand the meanings you attach to food and body size. Kano also devotes some time to exploring feelings about exercise and bringing it into your life in a pleasurable way. A unique feature of this book is a wonderful section for family and friends on what constitutes "support" for the person who is making peace with food and her body.

Susie Orbach, *Fat Is a Feminist Issue* (New York: Berkley, 1978). A classic on the psychological and cultural meanings of eating and weight. Particularly useful for women of any size who eat compulsively but does not acknowledge that there are people whose fat is not caused by psychological factors.

Janet Polivy and Peter Herman. *Breaking the Diet Habit* (New York: Basic Books, 1983). From the research team that pioneered the idea that dieting ("restrained eating") causes bingeing, good advice on how to stop dieting and eat normally.

Geneen Roth, *Breaking Free from Compulsive Eating* (Indianapolis: Bobbs-Merrill, 1984). The best all-around book on compulsive eating and how to stop. Roth also explores the self-defeating temptation to use exercise compulsively and the importance of approaching movement as a pleasurable activity.

Magazines and Newsletters of Interest

Ample Information. Published by Ample Opportunity, 5370 N.W. Roanoke Lane, Dept. R. 1, Portland, Oregon 97229. An informal, gutsy newsletter for fat women that's not afraid to ask difficult questions. Recent articles have been on the safety of aspartame (Nutrasweet); solving the problems of socially embarrassing situations; defining how fat is "fat"; fat and sexuality, and so forth. These folks also organize all kinds of sports and exercise classes, as well as discussion groups, clothing exchanges, and so on. Annual subscription rate is $10.

Ample Shopper Club Newsletter. Published bimonthly by Amplestuff, Ltd. Includes news articles and information relating to books and general merchandise for ample-sized people. A sample copy is available, along with the latest Amplestuff catalog and a $3 coupon, for $3. Write to: Amplestuff, Ltd., 1150 E. Market St., Charlottesville, VA 22901.

Big Beautiful Woman. Subtitled "The World's First Fashion Magazine for the Large-Size Woman," BBW presents colorful, lively clothes and articles of interest to larger women. For subscription information write to *Big Beautiful Women* Magazine, 5535 Balboa Boulevard, Suite 214, Encino, California 91316.

Breaking Free Newsletter. Published by Geneen Roth, author of *Feeding the Hungry Heart* and *Breaking Free* (cited above), this newsletter focuses on items of interest to people of all sizes struggling with compulsive eating. For information write to *Breaking Free,* P.O. Box 2852, Santa Cruz, California 95063.

The Grace-Full Eater. This quarterly newsletter is newly advertised as our paperback edition goes to press as a forum for "fighting fat oppression and making peace with food." $12.95 buys a year's subscription; write to 233 Forest Home Dr., Ithaca, NY 14850.

Hersize Newsletter. *Hersize* describes itself as a "weight prejudice action group" and this informal newsletter has movie and art reviews, discussions of the writings and political actions of members, and networking ideas. See "Organizations" and write to 223 Concord Ave., Toronto, Ontario. M6H 2P4 (Canada).

NAAFA Newsletter. Published monthly by the NATIONAL ASSOCIATION TO ADVANCE FAT ACCEPTANCE, INC. as a benefit of membership ($35 per year). Not a diet or weight-loss publication, it instead focuses on news about improving the quality of life for fat people through public education, research, advocacy, and support. Write to: NAAFA, Dept. GS, P.O. Box 188620, Sacramento, CA 95818; or call (916) 443-0303.

Radiance: The Magazine for Large Women. Published quarterly, this new journal on living a full life covers not only fashion but all topics of concern to larger women: exercise, self-esteem, finding health insurance—you name it. *Radiance* has grown beyond its San Francisco Bay Area roots into a nationwide magazine. For subscription information call (415) 482-0680; or write P.O. Box 31703, Oakland, California 94604; or look for *Radiance* at your local WALDENBOOK store.

Women's Sports and Fitness. Published as one activity of the Women's Sports Foundation, this is the first and only publication to respectfully and enthusiastically promote sports for women. Although it created grumbling among serious athletes when they added *Fitness* both to the title and the editorial content, the publication is dedicated to encouraging an active life-style for all women. Don't look for accepting attitudes about fat, but if you or your daughter needs encouragement or specific information about the sports you'd like to try, you may find it here. $14.95 per year. To subscribe call (800) 321-3333 or write to P.O. Box 3734, Escondido, California 92025.

Extra Special. Published bi-monthly. 65 Blandford Street, London, W1H3AJ, Tel (01) 402-9461.

Cachet. 9 Cavendish Square, London, W1M 9DD. Tel (01) 631-1801.

Additional Relevant Research

Paul Ernsberger and Paul Haskew. *Rethinking Obesity: An Alternative View of its Health Implications* (New York: Human Sciences Press, 1987). The authors review hundreds of studies in this exhaustive sweep of the epidemiological literature on obesity, and argue that the connection between obesity and ill health has been overstated and distorted. This is an authoritative review of one of the most hotly debated subjects in medicine, and a very useful source of hard data in arguments with the hard-headed.

Lisa Hunter, Ed. *Resource Guide: Friends Are Good Medicine,* Far West Laboratory for Educational Research and Development, San Francisco, California, 1982. Educational resources were prepared under a contract with the California Department of Mental Health, Mental Health Promotion Branch. The materials provide an overview of research conducted on the mental and physical health benefits of social support and are the basis for an ongoing statewide mental health promotion educational campaign. Relevant data referenced in chapter one: Berkman, L. F., and Syme, L. (1979), "Social Networks, Host Resistance, and Mortality: A Nine-Year Study of Alameda County Residents." American Journal of *Epidemiology 109 (2)*: pages 186-204. Also see Brown, G. W., Bahrolchin, M. N. and Harris, T., "Social Class and Psychiatric Disturbance Among Women in an Urban Population." *Sociology 9,* 1975.

Phoebe Jones. Survey report from the North American Network of Women Runners, collected in "Resources for Women's Fitness and Sports" (contained in preconferenced material prepared for *The New Agenda: The Future of Women and Sports,* Washington D.C., 1983.) This and a wide variety of additional research data relative to the participation of women in sports can be obtained from the Women's Sports Foundation, New York, New York.

Robert Ornstein, Ph.D. and David Sobel, M.D. *Healthy Pleasures* (New York: Addison Wesley, 1989). Finally, a book based on common sense, backed by abundant research data, that says you don't have to kill yourself to save your life. Emphasizing the health benefits of pleasurable pursuits, the authors debunk many longstanding myths, including those about weight.

Appendix II

Activities and Exercise Classes

(By State)

(Some listings, such as "Women at Large," and "Dana's Full Figure Salon," are budding franchise operations that may have additional locations nationwide. Check with their headquarters for current information. Appearance on this list does not imply the authors' recommendation.)

Nationwide

Check your local YMCA for their re-entry exercise program for beginners called "The Y's Way to Fitness." Many Y's also have an Aqua-Aerobics program to work out in the pool. these are standardized programs offered across the country, and while they are not designed exclusively for large women, you might find they meet your needs better than the typical aerobics class.

Alaska

Anchorage Women at Large
907 E. Dowling Road, Suite 30
Anchorage, AK 99518
(907) 562-6252

Arizona

Phoenix Women at Large
5140 W. Peoria, Suite 5
Glendale, AZ 85301
(602) 486-2886

California

The Big Splash
San Francisco, CA
(415) 237-3978 (Jan)
(415) 285-1769 (Miriam)

Bodymoves Workout Studio
1283 Camino Del Rio South
San Diego, CA 92108
(619) 297-9959

Curves Unlimited: Advocacy of
Health and Fitness for Large
People
Gail Johnson, Personal Fitness
Instructor
Walnut Creek, CA
(415) 945-8891

Dance and Movement for Big,
Beautiful Bodies
Sharon Page-Ritchie
Oakland YWCA
Oakland, CA
(415) 531-9267

El Cajon Women at Large
735 Jamacha Road
El Cajon, CA 92019
(619) 441-8211

Fremont Women at Large
Flex Fitness Center
41899 Albrae Street
Fremont, CA 04538
(415) 490-1843

The Image as Given
Beginning Jazz and Movement Class
Los Angeles Area
Judith Parker, Ph.D.
(213) 281-1961

Making Waves
2423 Douglas St.
San Pablo, CA 94806
(415) 237-3978 (Jan)

Upland Women at Large
1937 W. 11th Street, Unit E
Upland, CA 91786
(714) 949-1408

Colorado

Positively More
Pat Moore
Fitness Department Assistant
South Suburban Parks & Recreation
District
6315 South University Blvd
Littleton, CO 80121
(303) 798-2476, ext. 141
(303) 795-5933 home

Thornton Women at Large
690 W. 84th Avenue
Thornton, CO 80221
(303) 426-6981

Connecticut

Waterford Women at Large
Crossroads Center
167 Parkway North
Waterford, CT 06385
(203) 437-1301

Florida

Largo Women at Large
3690 East Bay Drive, Suite L
Largo, FL 34641
(813) 536-2551

Georgia

Atlanta Women at Large
11235 Alpharetta Highway, Suite 101
Rosewell, GA 30076
(404) 751-9188

Idaho

Blackfoot Women at Large
Riverside Plaza
Blackfoot, ID 83221
(208) 785-5292

Maryland

Gaithersburg Women at Large
18228 Flower Hill Way
Gaithersburg, MD 20879
(301) 670-1943

Minnesota

Dance Fun for Large Women
5308 Chateau Place
Minneapolis, MN
55417
(612) 722-0722

Panda's
11503 K-Tel Drive
Minnetonka, MN
55343
(612) 935-5354

St. Louis Park Women at Large
5340 Cedar Lake Road
St. Louis Park, MN 55416
(612) 541-0671

Women's Aerobics Plus
4201 Minnetonka Blvd
St. Louis Park, MN 55416
(612) 926-5149
(612) 926-6561

Nevada

Reno Women at Large
1180 West 4th Street
Reno, NV 89503
(702) 323-3311

New York

Bourne Exercise Studio
One Chase Road
Scarsdale, NY 10583
(914) 472-4144

Jan Stritzler (individual exercise
trainer)
Fitness Designs
501 East 85th Street, #2B
New York, NY 10028

Lisa Swerdlow
The Smart Move
131 West 72nd Street
New York, NY 10023
(212) 260-1520

North Carolina

Easy Does It
YWCA of Wake County
1012 Oberlin Road
Raleigh, NC 27605
(919) 828-3205

Oregon

Ample Opportunity
5370 N.W. Roanoke Lane
Portland, OR 97229
(503) 645-0497
(Belly Dance; Tai Chi classes;
swimming, volleyball, Sunday walks,
cross-country skiing, weekend
canoeing)

Pennsylvania

Aerobics in Moderation
Mid-City YWCA
2027 Chestnut Street
Philadelphia, PA 19103
(215) 564-3430

Big, Beautiful, and Fit
Frankford YWCA
Arrott and Leiper Streets
Philadelphia, PA 19124
(215) 831-9500

Greensburg Women at Large
Greensburg Shopping Center
East Pittsburgh Street
Greensburg, PA 15601
(412) 837-8103

Shippenville Women at Large
P.O. Box 316
Second Street
Shippenville, PA 16254
(814) 782-6237

Texas

Midland Women at Large
Mesa Verde Shopping Center
2215 N. Midland, Suite 4-D
Midland, TX 79707
(915) 697-5558

Richardson Women at Large
1600 N. Plano Road, Suite 800
Richardson, TX 75081
(214) 644-2226

Virginia

Extrasize
Ruth Crane
Norfolk, VA
(804) 473-8084

Washington

Chris Zagelow Patterson
IDEA Fitness Consultant
Walla Walla, WA
(509) 529-0346

Spokane Women at Large
W. 3330 Central
Spokane, WA 99204
(509) 327-6492

Women at Large
1020 South 48th Avenue
Yakima, WA 98908
(509) 965-0115

Wisconsin

Brown Deer Women at Large
4425 W. Bradley
Brown Deer, WI 53223
(414) 354-2774

Canada

Sally Olson
Grand Size Fitness
Vancouver Area
(206) 574-5306

Edmonton #1 Women at Large
#212 8915 51 Avenue
Edmonton, AB, Canada
(403) 465-2923

Edmonton #2 Women at Large
10114 175th Street
Edmonton, AB, Canada
(403) 484-9824

Edmonton #3 Women at Large
Box 3152
Edmonton, AB, Canada
(403) 986-5544

Kamloops Women at Large
12-1425 Cariboo Place
Kamloops, BC, Canada
(604) 828-1211

Victoria Women at Large
1044 Fort Street
Victoria, BC, Canada
(604) 389-1442

Great Britain

Big Women Swim
Hackney Women's Centre
20 Dalston Lane
London, E9
(01) 986-0840

Want to Play Net Ball, Rounders
London Area
Doreen
(01) 659-8843

Organizations

Ample Information
5370 N.W. Roanoke Lane
Portland, OR 97229
(503) 645-0497

This active group based in Portland published a newsletter and organizes all kinds of social, educational, and sporting activities for large women.

Big City Woman
Ms. Cecile Dare
4485 Park Blvd.
San Diego, CA
(619) 692-3855

A support group which provides networking origination for larger-sized business and professional women.

Fat Lip Reader's Theater
P.O. Box 7717
Berkeley, CA 94707

Fat Lip Reader's Theater, 16 "fat, feisty women speaking, acting and singing about being fat in America in the 80s" now have a 30 minute videotape, "Nothing to Lose," so that audiences beyond the San Francisco Bay Area can enjoy their groundbreaking work.

HERSIZE: A Weight Prejudice Action Group
222 Concord Avenue
Toronto, Ontario M6H 2P4

This wonderful Canadian group publishes a newsletter (see "Newsletters/Magazines") and a resource guide, sponsors workshops, makes media presentations, and developed a slide show on weight obsession. Membership is a well-spend $25.

Largely Positive
Carol Johnson
5531 N. Navaho Avenue
Milwaukee, WI 53217
(414) 964-2804

This is an organization hoping to launch a number of different events, including workshops, self-esteem groups and movement/exercise classes.

Model Mugging of Monterey
801 Lighthouse Avenue
Monterey, CA 93940
(408) 646-5425

Model Mugging is a unique self-defense course for women. Male instructors wear padding so that students can practice using their full strength against an assailant, in scenarios that are highly realistic and with the expert coaching of a female instructor. There are many California locations as well as a growing number across the nation.

National Association to Advance Fat Acceptance, Inc. (NAAFA)
Department GS
P.O. Box 188620
Sacramento, CA 95818
(916) 443-0303

NAAFA has been educating and working for size acceptance since 1969, achieving impressive legal, medical, and personal victories for large people. There are over 35 chapters in the United States and Canada. See listing under "Magazines/Newsletters."

Women's Health and Reproductive Rights Information Centre
52 Featherstone Street
London EC1H 8RT

Information relating to large women and all aspects of health.

Exercise Videos
Designed Specifically for Large Women.

Please note: The authors do not endorse particular videos. We thank Gail Johnston and Alice Ansfield for allowing us to reprint an adaptation of Gail's spring 1989 article in *Radiance Magazine,* which reviews many of the following videos.

Big on Fitness $24.95 video
(800) 999-4952   tax/shipping charges not
available

Danasize Video $49.95 video
15447 SE 9th St.   3.95 tax (WA residents only)
Bellevue, WA 98007   3.00 shipping/handling

Feel Beautiful $39.95 video
B. R. Anderson Enterprises 2.40 tax (MN residents only)
5308 Chateau Place   2.95 postage/handling

Idrea Says "Yes You Can" $24.95 video
Two Lipps Video   2.00 shipping/handling
(800) 87-IDREA

In Grand Form $29.95, complete
Grand Form Enterprises Ltd.
P.O. Box 87000
North Vancouver, BC V7L 4P6
(604) 984-9435

Just Move $24.95 video
D. P. Moves   4.00 postage/handling
P.O. Box 5201
San Jose, CA 95150-5201
(408) 241-1510

Light on Your Feet $29.99 video
P.O. Box 1841   3.00 shipping/handling
Hyattsville, MD 20782

Jean Rosenbaum, M.D. $49.95 video
P.O. Box 401   2.00 handling
Durango, CO 81301
(303) 247-4109

Women At Large—Breakout $29.95 video
1020 South 48th Ave.   3.00 shipping/handling
Yakima, WA 98908
(800) 346-6134

Women In Motion—An Odyssey $19.95 video
Pamela Gurnick, M.D.   3.00 shipping/handling
Big Tape Enterprises
P.O. Box 19000
Alexandria, VA 22320
(800) 582-2000

Women On the Move
by Gail Johnston
(Article updated and reprinted with permission from *Radiance* Magazine, Spring 1989.)

There is certainly good news for you on the exercise video front. More and more videos are being created for large women with instructors and back-up students who are also large women.

BUT, I'm still waiting for the video that I can recommend to you without modification, without reservation, without dying of embarassment. Each of the videos I've reviewed receives an un- equivocal A for effort: It is exceedingly difficult and expensive to produce a video, and sponsor dollars are not as available to these "specialty market" videos. When I read other reviews of these "spe- cialty" videos, they seem to give A's to all of the videos even when they're not deserving of them. It's as if they're saying "Isn't it sweet that those fat ladies are exercising. The video doesn't need to be that great because the audience isn't as discriminating."

So you may think my reviews have a more critical eye than other video reviews. That's because I believe you have a right to expect an attractive set, a competent instructor demonstrating safe exercises, back-up people who are doing the exercises properly, and a motivat- ing workout presented with enthusiasm.

So far, my dream exercise video is:
Set: "Women at Large"
Music: "Sweatin to the Oldies"
Introduction: Jody Sandler of "In Grand Form"
Instructor: Idrea ("Idrea says Yes You Can")
Back-Up:Rosezella Canty-Letsome ("Light on Your Feet") and Nel- lie Petersen ("Just Move")

Big on Fitness
with Kathy Bell
Music Style: light jazz or new age, mostly in background
Movement style: easy rhythmical, athletic

After reading a rave review of this video in a fitness magazine, I couldn't wait to tear the wrapper off my own copy. Kathy and her team of four, all large women, lead you through a 50-minute com- plete workout which includes low-impact aerobics, lower body strengthening and stretching. The program is structured so that you can exercise with any or all of the segments.

The "Big on Fitness" concept was developed by Jack Kirkham of the Oakway Spa in Eugene, OR, based on interviews with physicians and large women. The focus is on starting an activity plan rather than losing weight. Aside from a few contradictory exercises (e.g., knee rolls for sides of the waist, snapping/locking the knees), the exercises themselves are trustworthy.

But we have an enormously high boredom factor here. Kathy didn't smile at me once, and the bulk of what she said to me was "Keep breathing." and "4-3-2-1." The women in the background look like exercising was the last thing they wanted to be doing that day. The music wasn't even loud enough to divert my attention from the monotone quality of the workout.

This well-intentioned exercise program was on target with its goals: emphasizing self-esteem and a gradual development of your fitness skills. But it's just not FUN! And when exercise isn't fun, it feels like work. And when exercise feels like work, I don't do it.

Danasize
with Lee Dana
Music style: jazz, lots of brass
Movement style: gym class

Hitting the market in 1985, *Danasize* was one of the first exercise videos for, by and starring large women. Two workouts are included on this tape: a 45-minute beginner level and a 45-minute advanced level. Lee Dana doesn't do much exercising herself; she stands on the edge of the tiny room trying to offer individual attention to her six students without getting hit by a wayward arm or leg. *Danasize,* a forerunner of size acceptance in fitness, is the unfortunate victim of time and scientific advancement. The workout includes lots of un-supported forward flexion, ballistic movement, straight leg sit-ups (tough on the back) and no aerobics. Dana is wonderful, sincere, committed—imagine the obstacles she had to overcome to get her concept on tape and into distribution. I wish her studio in Washington were still open so she would be inspired to create *Danasize II.* Still, I can't recommend this video because so many of the exercises are either ineffective or so dangerous that your greatest exertion would be spent in trying to invent modifications for the movements.

Feel Beautiful
with Barbara Anderson
Music style: mostly light piano, some country
Movement style: nonrhythmical

Barbara's newly revised introduction for *Feel Beautiful* is a gentle, motivational message shot with a hand-held camera in a backyard, home-movie style. Her manner is warm and compassionate, and she is subtle in conveying the educational information so important for first-timers. The video has three components: (1) Calisthenics and aerobics, (2) relaxation, and (3) mental conditioning.

The informal approach of "showing genuine people having fun while working together to build healthy bodies and healthy minds" didn't work for me. I was extremely uncomfortable with the fact that Barbara and the two women behind her (one of whom shared the role of instructor) demonstrated mostly unsafe exercises, and stopped movement between aerobic songs to review upcoming exercises. They appeared to have no idea what they were doing. In fact, as they continued to botch the exercises and ignore the musical beat, I started feeling clumsy myself and, even worse, distrustful of their knowledge. Including a relaxation segment was a lovely idea, but it is so hard to hear Barbara's voice over the music that relaxation can only occur if you ignore her voice.

Barbara promotes herself as a certified instructor, but her forte is obviously more in the area of mental conditioning than physical. Let her affirmations become a part of your present. Let her exercises become part of your past.

Idrea Says "Yes You Can"
with Idrea
Music style: combination of lively aerobic beat and jazz
Movement style: rhythmical and athletic

This exercise video was just released in March and it is, without question, my top choice for the all-around safe, fun, total body workout. Idrea is the picture of health—strong, vibrant, body-confident. There is nothing shy or subtle about her. Look beyond her weight-loss message and you'll see a proud, sexy, large woman (with a bent for comedy) who likes to "strut her stuff" and wants you to do the same. Her exercise selections are sound, her alignment is impeccable, and her instruction is direct, if not boisterous.

To say Idrea enjoys teaching is an understatement. The "freestyle" (do whatever you want to do) portion of aerobics is a nice reminder that movement is a gift you can give yourself whenever the spirit (or a good song) inspires you. By means of a screen inset (a smaller version of the big screen that is set off in a corner), the option is open to do the strengthening exercises standing rather than seated on the floor.

This one-hour video is great for all fitness levels. Adaptations for the various exercises are offered throughout, so listen for them. Okay, so the cameras get a little artsy, and the inset boxes are a little small, and the weight loss directives are a little pushy: I still love it.

**In Grand Form
with Jody Sandler**
Music style: jazz with brass (some sassy) and one song with country flavor
Movement style: rhythmical, slightly dancy

I didn't want to like this video because it had such a down-home look, not contemporary enough for my "nouvelle fitnesse" tastes. But it slowly won me over due almost entirely to the 41-year-old instructor, Jody, who is just so warm and likeable.

The video has its strongest appeal for brand new exercisers who want to get a feel for aerobics-type movement in the security of their own home. For the first eight minutes, you'll receive a slow, simple explanation of "the basics": shoes, water, how to take heart rate and find your target heart rate range, etc. After you learn the information, you can skip that part of the video and concentrate on the exercises.

Before you even begin, Jody also reviews the basic movements you'll be doing later in the aerobics section. This way, you won't be trying to master the steps while you're trying to get your heart rate up. So you can feel smooth and polished rather than clumsy on your first time through. (This workout also proves that simple exercises can still be interesting.)

There is, however, one confusing aspect to this video: Jody and her supporting talent, representing all age levels, demonstrate the exercises at three different intensity levels. A good idea, but you find yourself looking at each of them wondering what to do next. Stick with Jody. And in the warm-up, there's one exercise that involves a reach to the ceiling, then to the hips, then to the floor. Nix the floor reach—it's tough on the back. Also in the warm-up and cool-down is a stretch that asks you to balance on one leg; until you get the hang of it, use the wall or a chair for support.

I recommend this video for absolute beginners who care more about surviving their first exercise experiences than learning how exercise will lower their blood pressure. But I also think you'll graduate to your next video fairly quickly.

Just Move
with Nellie Petersen
Music style: standard aerobic music
Movement style: Non-dancy, straightforward exercise

Nellie's message to her viewers is "I've been working out since I was 17—I may not look like a model but I move with grace and control. Exercise affords me the energy to lead an active life . . . The importance of JUST MOVE is to exercise whether trying to lose weight or not." And Nellie is right! Her energy, strength and grace make her a good role model for other large women.

Unfortunately, her video advisors let her down. To be effective, an exercise video must have a certain amount of entertainment value, and the exercisers must see the importance of their roles as performers. "Just Move" does an injustice to Nellie's spirit, talent and (I am guessing) philosophy by falling short in the areas of camera work and technical and talent direction.

Let's start with the camera work. In order to follow along with an exercise video, you must be able to see what the instructor is doing. Focusing on a face when the feet are changing position doesn't help the viewer learn the routine. And the camera should always be on individuals who can do the exercise correctly so that you can feel confident following any of the people you see.

While the majority of exercises are safe, there are a few that need modification: any leaning forward or to the side should be preceded by at least one hand for support; when you lie on your side doing leg lifts, don't bring your legs so far forward that your body forms an "L". (This video also utilizes the confusing three-ability-level demonstration of exercises—so follow Nellie.)

I would guess that Nellie's live exercise classes are a real hoot—she just seems to have that kind of flair. I especially like it when she says "There's nothing wrong with stopping" because that's a valuable instructor cue left out of most exercise videos (and classes!). But her personality is never revealed in this video. In fact, her only smiles are on the video box. Somebody should have said "Put the music on, and let her rip." She might have seemed less rigid. And you might feel more motivated to put the video in your VCR.

Light on Your Feet
with Rosezella Canty-Letsome
Music style: lively jazz, not boring at all
Movement style: some dancy, some rhythmical

This 60-minute workout is another vintage 1985 model. Despite the inclusion of an aerobics segment, the movements are still obsolete: ballistic, fast, unsupported forward flexion, straight leg sit-ups and the deadly hurdler's stretch. The majority of exercises show little of the reverence for the spine that is essential for a safe workout. Again, it's no one's fault: research can outdate a video in the same month it hits the video stores.

I do, however, recommend that you watch (no following along, please) for a boost of motivational oom-pah-pah! Rosezella is the personification of joy in movement. A party is going on in this woman's body and we've all been invited to join the celebration. I smiled from beginning to end. At the end of the arm section, Rosezella stretches with the words "Hug yourself. Love yourself." It's like the best scene from an Academy Award movie—you'll want to watch it over and over. The six back-ups vary in age and size and are proof positive that fitness is for every body.

Sweatin to the Oldies
with Richard Simmons
Music style: fifties tunes
Movement style: mostly dancy, some dramatic interpretation

I say "Richard Simmons," and you probably say, "No, thank you. He doesn't like me the way I am. He wants me to be thin." Meet the new Richard. His message is still weight loss, but you won't hear those words even once on this video.

What will you hear? Bruce Willis's band—Live—playing blast-from-past favorites at a mock high school reunion for Richard and his "school chums," who represent all sizes and fitness abilities. This aerobics-only video (with complete warm-up and cool-down) has the most surprising effect on everyone who exercises with it: They smile, they reminisce, they sing, they dance, they do silly movements to songs like "It's My Party," *and* they keep putting the video back in the VCR day after day because it's so much fun.

No one is having more fun than Richard, as he lives out his exercise fantasy in front of our eyes. The video is short on instruction, but Richard's alignment is on the money, at least from his knees up. A self-proclaimed flatfooter, Richard's feet are not able to cooperate with proper foot/knee placement, so let the feet of those to his immediate left or right be your guide. The overhead camera angles for "Ain't No Mountain High Enough" are somewhat distracting to the flow of the movement, but I doubt you'll care much because you'll be living out your own "Peggy Sue" fantasy.

Women at Large-Breakout
with Sharlyne Powell and Sharon McConnell
Music style: aerobic beat with lots of brass
Movement style: part dancy, part rhythmical

The Women at Large concept has attracted a considerable amount of media attention. With the financial support of Fitting Pretty Pantyhose, Sharlyne and Sharon, owners of the Women at Large fitness franchise, created the *Women at Large—Breakout* exercise video. The set is gorgeous, the instructors and students exude good health, the movements are all well-rehearsed, and the message of size acceptance is unmistakably clear.

What a disappointment that the exercises being demonstrated leave so much to be desired in safety and effectiveness: locked knees, hyperextension of the neck, joint snapping, fast and jerky movements, and an unforgivable amount of unsupported forward flexion for a video so recently released. They should have known better. These are the kinds of movements that leave you feeling sore the next day, or worse. Only an expert in alignment modifications would be able to make the number of exercise adaptations to make these exercises worthwhile—slowing down, softening knees, adding support, protecting the joints, and so on.

Skip over the exercise segment and go directly to the end of the video to hear heartfelt motivational stories from large women who have broken through exercise barriers and come out on the winning side. They'll take you through an emotional workout that will leave you feeling energized, high on exercise and standing on your chair applauding.

Women in Motion—An Odyssey
with Peggy Farrell and Mark Bergel
Music style: classical with an aerobic beat
Movement style: nondancy, straight-forward exercise

Three female physicians provided medical supervision for this specially designed "odyssey" for large women. As a result, the medical bias is strongly present. The gloom and doom message: "If you are obese, that is, 50 pounds overweight or greater you are at risk for a wide range of medical problems." And the enclosed Fact Sheet lists the potential problems. Threats have never been successful in motivating me to exercise.

The video opens on Dr. Gurnick, one of the medical directors, discussing the importance of safe exercise with Peggy and Mark in a manner that is as light-hearted as "Apocalypse Now." Peggy, whose voice becomes raw as the workout progresses, and Mark, whose style is warm and supportive, team-teach the class, share the cueing, and work with each of the students independently.

The workout is safe for the entry level exerciser, but is often difficult to follow because the music does not match the movement and because the camera seems uncertain which of the five people to follow at any given moment. What disturbs me the most, however, is that they don't seem to include me, the home exerciser, in the workout. Peggy and Mark even turn their back to the camera for the stretches at the end.

There's a nice quickie explanation on proper use of the rowing machine and the stationary bike. This video, which obviously came straight from the hearts of three caring physicians, just missed its target. They intend to produce more, and will hopefully learn from this experience.

Clothing Suppliers and Catalogues

Below we report on Variety Catalogues, General Clothing Catalogues, Specialty Clothing Catalogues, Suppliers, and Clothing Stores with mail order services. Following this, our researcher Robin Hopkins describes the dancewear in more detail. In a third and final section, we report on sewing resources (patterns, fabrics, and references).

A note on sizes: Some manufacturers size their clothing by waist or hip measurement in inches; others by dress size; others by blouse size. You might be unfamiliar with the "x" sizes (1x, 2x, 3x, 4x, 5x): this is the sizing system that some manufacturers of large size clothing use to distinguish it from average size clothing.

Variety Catalogues

Amplestuff Catalogue **$3.00**
Amplestuff, Ltd.
Dept. GS
1150 E. Market St.
Charlottesville, VA 22901

Full Figure Fashion Directory **$10.00**
Shopping by Mail
Cathy Cooper
23 E. 10th St. #304
Dept. GS
New York, NY 10003

General Clothing Catalogues

Sue Brett
P.O. Box 8301
Indianapolis, IN 46283-8301
  Sweats, activewear, bras dancewear,
  swimsuits

Lane Bryant
P.O. Box 7201
Indianapolis, IN 46207-7201
  Sweats, activewear, bras, dancewear,
  swimsuits

For You (Spiegel)
Katie Lavins
1515 W. 224th St.
Oakbrook, IL
60521
  Varies with season

L'Eggs
Just My Size
P.O. Box 6000
Rural Hall, NC 27098
  Sweats, dancewear

Nancy's Choice
P.O. Box 7201
Indianapolis, IN 46207-7201
  (Info not available)

Regalia (formerly Pueblo Traders)
Palo Verde at 33rd St.
P.O. Box 27800-7800
Tucson, AZ 85726
  Activewear, bras, swimsuits

Roaman's
P.O. Box 8301
Indianapolis, IN 46283-8301
  Sweats, activewear, bras, dancewear,
  swimsuits

Silhouettes
Dept. EM-2032 Building #70
Hanover, PA 17333
  Sweats

Specialty Catalogues

Big Stitches
by Jan
2423 Douglas St.
San Pablo, CA 94806
(415) 237-3978
  Custom-made swimsuits sized 36–70+

Body by Ruben
17109 Locust Dr.
Hazelcrest, IL 60429
(312) 335-0933
  Dancewear to 4x

Full Bloom
185 S. Pearl
Denver, CO 80209
  T-shirts, sweats 2x–9x

Making It Big
P.O. Box 203
Cotati, CA 94928
  Natural Fiber Sportswear, including
  supersize

Schatzi Designs
1283 Blvd. Way
Walnut Creek, CA 94595
  Exercise Wear to 3x

Upscale Sweats
Peggy Lutz Design
P.O. Box 170665
San Francisco, CA 94117
  50% Cotton Sweats, including supersize

Women at Large
1020 S. 48th Ave.
Yakima, WA 98908
  Exercise Wear

Suppliers

Advantage
150 W. Jefferson Blvd.
Los Angeles, CA 9007
  Dancewear

Custom Wardrobe Design
Karen Louise Maley
7777 Fay Avenue, Suite K-273
La Jolla, CA 92037
(619) 272-3301

Danskin Plus
350 Fifth Ave.
New York, NY 10018
(717) 846-4874
  Dancewear

Formfit Rogers
12 W. 27th St.
NY, NY 10001
(212) 688-3900
  Bras

Great Gal
1407 Broadway #1216
NY, NY 10018
  Activewear

Grid Sports
5801 Mariemont
Cincinnati, OH 45227
(513) 271-3400
  (Elastic support band worn over bra)

Hersey Custom Shoe Co.
RFD #3, Box 7390
Farmington, ME 04938
(207) 778-3103
  Walking and running shoes to
  15 EEEEEE

International Playtex
215 College Rd.
P.O. Box 728
Paramus NJ 07652
  Bras

Lotsa Lottie
5 Town and Country Village,
Suite 738
San Jose, CA 95128
(408) 287-8186
    "Whimsical Play Clothes": Sweats, T's

Parklane
1540 Union Turnpike
N. Hyde Park, NJ 11040
(516) 328-7400
    Dancewear to 4x

Rainbeau Outlet
300 4th St.
San Francisco, CA 94107
(415) 777-9786
    Dancewear

Schatzi Designs
1283 Blvd Way
Walnut Creek, CA 94595
(415) 943-1199
    Dancewear

Special Events by
Extra Sportswear
1407 Broadway
NY, NY 10018
(212) 239-0400
    Sweats

Great Britain

Above Average
35 Market Street,
Loughborough,
Leics, LE 11 3ER.
Tel (0509) 264037

Annabel
High Street,
Bishops Waltham,
Southampton,
Hants, SO3 1AA.
Tel (04893) 3645

Anne's Fashions
11 North Methven Street,
Perth,
Tayside, PH1 5PN.
Tel (0738) 22884

Aquarius
39–41 Wellington Road,
Ashton,
Preston,
Lancs, PR2 1BU
Tel (0772) 728 069

The Ballroom
Bayshill Lodge,
Montpeller,
Cheltenham,
Glos, GL50 1ST Y

The Base
55 Monmouth Street,
Covent Garden,
London, WC2H 9DG.
Tel (01) 240 8914.

Big Clothes
81A Boundary Road,
London, NW8.
Tel (01) 722 1127.

Big Ideas
5 Newtown Road,
Bishops
Stortford,
Herts, CM23 2DW.
Tel (0279) 506 766.

Big Sister
(mail order)
4 St. John's Crescent,
Canton, Cardiff, CF5 1NX.
Tel (0222) 24249.

Beech Tree
Raglan Street,
Halifax, HX1 5QX.
Tel (0422) 65204.
 Sixteen shops and mail
 order.

Bloyle
40 Sloane Street,
London, SW1X 9LP.
Tel (01) 245 9806.

Buy and Large
4 Holbein Place,
Sloane Square,
London, SW1W 8NP.
Tel (01) 730 6534.

Claire Mont
18 Northgate,
Basildon,
Shipley,
West Yorkshire, BD17 6JX.
Tel (0274) 586 010.

Diana Lucy
54 Spring Gardens,
Buxton,
Derbyshire.
(0298) 5687.

Dickins and Jones
224 Regent Street,
London, W1A 1DB.
(01) 734 7070.

Dressing Up
10 Maryport Road,
Lady Mary Estate,
Cardiff, CF2 5JX.
Tel (0222) 757 048.

Escorpion
296 Station Road,
Harrow,
Middx, HA1 2DX.
Tel (0483) 898 222.

Evans Collections
Evans Press Office,
214 Oxford Street,
London, W1N 9DF.
Tel (01) 636 8040.

Evelyn Clare
627 Watford Way,
Mill Hill,
London, NW7 3JN.
Tel (01) 959 5056.

Extra Elegance
10 Lindow Parade,
Off Capel Lane,
Wilmslow,
Ches, SK9 5JL.
Tel (0625) 525 402.

The Extra Inch
16 William Street,
West End,
Edinburgh, EH3 7NH.
Tel (031) 226 3303.

Fabriani
36 Sere Road,
Clarkston,
Glasgow, G76 7QF.
Tel (041) 638 4441.

Feathers
155 High Street,
Hurstpierpoint,
Hassocks,
West Sussex, BN6 9PU.
Tel (0273) 83468.

Fine Figures
9 The Precinct,
High Road,
Broxbourne,
Herts, EN10 7HY.
Tel (0992) 44297.

Forgotten Woman
275 High Road,
Loughton,
Essex, IG10 1AH.
Tel (01) 508 4654.

Gabe Gowns
233 Baker Street,
London, NW1 6XE.
Tel (01) 935 0217.

Generosity
14a George Street,
St Albans,
Herts, AL3 4ER.
Tel (0727) 32095.

Harringtons
129 The Broadway,
Mill Hill,
London, NW 7 4RN.
Tel (01) 959 2312.

Impact
59 Station Road,
Edgeware,
Middx, HA8 7HX.
Tel (01) 951 1552.

Maggie of Warlingham
20 The Green,
Warlingham,
Surrey, CR3 9NA.
Tel (0883) 23594.

Monica Flynn
11/12 Halkin Arcade,
Motcombe Street,
London, SW1X 8JT.
Tel (01) 245 9896.

One of Gillies
Liantrithyd,
Cowbridge,
South Glamorgan, CF7
7UB.
Tel (04468) 357.

Pat Atkinson
1/3 Cavendish Street,
Ulverston,
Cumbria, LA12 7AD.
Tel (0229) 5466.

Patricia's
103 High Street,
Chislehurst,
Kent, BR7 5AN.
Tel (01) 467 1800.

Pearson's
Upper Parliament Street,
Nottingham.
Tel (0602) 475 761.

Rendezvous
17 The Parade,
St Mary's Place,
Shrewsbury,
Salop, SY1.
Tel (0742) 68325.

Rita Fashions
6 Turnpike Parade,
Green Lanes,
London, N15 3EA.
Tel (01) 888 6234.

Rosie Dees Designs
Church Finance House,
Radley Road Industrial
Estate,
Abingdon,
Oxfordshire, OX14 3SE.
Tel (0235) 34760.

Sassa
76 Rochester Row,
Victoria,
London, SW1P 1JU.
Tel 01 834 2266.

Secret Lady
Unit K13, Regent Arcade,
Cheltenham,
Glos, GL50 1JZ.
Tel (0242) 671 757.

Three Jay
9 The Precinct,
East Hoathly,
East Sussex, BN8 6DP.
Tel (0992) 442 974.

Xelle
51 Dorset Street,
London, W1H 3FA.
Tel (01) 935 5352.

Xtra
115a Golders Green Road,
London, NW11 8HR.
Tel (01) 455 7870.

Lingerie and Nightwear

Can-Can
188 Grays Inn Road,
London, WC1X 8EW.
Tel (01) 833 3531.

Dans-Ez
35 Sloane Gardens,
London, SW1W 8EB.
Tel (01) 730 9281.

Delia Marketin
24 Craven Park Road,
London, NW10 4AB.
Tel (01) 965 8707.

Rigby and Peller
2 Hans Road,
Knightsbridge,
London, SW3 1RX.
Tel (01) 589 9293.

Leotards

Carita House
London Road,
Stapely,
Nantwich,
Cheshire, CW5 7LJ.
Tel (0270) 627 722.

Clothing Stores with Mail Order Services

Abundance
3870 24th St.
San Francisco, CA 94114
(415) 550-8811
    Aerobic gear sized 14–26

Bentley's
2122 Shattuck Ave.
Berkeley, CA 94704
(415) 843-7595
    Dancewear, specifically Danskin Plus sized
14–29

Our researcher Robin Hopkins comments on the above brands:

Many people find sweats, shorts, and T-shirts comfortable for dance or exercise class, but leotards and tights are my favorite activewear. Why? They are less cumbersome; you can see your body's outlines and easily tell whether you are properly aligned; and they are cooler in the summer and warmer in the winter. But mostly they make me feel like a dancer!

Unfortunately, there appear to be only a few companies making leotards and tights in large sizes. If you are a size 14–20 you may be able to wear a standard "extra large," carried in most department, hosiery, or dancewear stores.

Otherwise, the following companies (for which addresses and/ or telephone numbers were given in the preceding chart) make large-size dancewear:

Advantage is Richard Simmons' line of tights and leotards in a variety of soft pastels and primary colors. He uses a high-quality cotton lycra fabric that is soft on the skin. The leotards "blouse" at the waist. Advantage can be found in many department stores.

Danskin Plus has expanded into an exciting, high-quality line. Although it is on the expensive side ($45 for a leotard), it is being carried in both dancewear stores and large-size stores and is therefore the most accessible large-size dancewear on the market. Given Danskin's longevity, it should be available for the foreseeable future.

Invitation to the Dance is a new line offering superb fit and quality due to the 4-way stretch Lycra fabric used. The feeling of having a "second skin" that firmly supports and allows unlimited range of motion is heavenly.

Lane Bryant, Sue Brett, and Roaman's have all carried the same line of dancewear in their catalogs recently. The fabric is a nylon/ polyester blend that is reasonably priced, but even the 3x (55–62″ hips) ran a little small.

Parklane Hosiery, with stores nationwide, carries a 1x–3x line in some stores. At the time of compiling this list, the Parklane representative reported that the line was not doing well and there were doubts about expanding it. But the things I have purchased fit well and ranged in price depending on fabric and snazziness.

Schatzi Designs manufactures a line of large-size as well as standard size dancewear, and the owner believes the large woman deserves the same options as the average-sized woman. Her leotards have high-cut French legs and are made of rich colors and prints. She has also begun making large-size unitards, which are tights and leotard in one. All items are available by mail. Sizes run from 1x to 3x and are on the smaller side. Her prices may seem high at first, but everything I have bought has worn well and is of high quality materials and workmanship. My wildest outfits come from Schatzi!

Spiegel's FOR YOU Catalogue carries a variety of dancewear, generally a "tank" style leotard in great primary colors, but only to a size 2XL (40–42). The fabric is a combination of polyester/cotton/lycra spandex knit. Tights are nylon/lycra spandex knit. Leotards have high-cut legs, great for both looks and freedom of movement.

Women-At-Large is an exercise studio in Yakima, Washington, which manufactures its own dancewear. Most of their styles have puffed sleeves. They also carry a large-size unitard. It comes in two-tone fabric, often a solid fabric on the bottom and print on the top. They have a great brochure and a range of sizes (12–24) that includes a tall size.

The range of shoes is staggering. Among my We Dance classmates, there is little consensus about which brand is the best, since everyone seems to prefer a different one. As a general tip, if you have wide feet, try men's athletic shoes, Hersey's mail order (listed in the preceding chart), or a specialty store carrying wider shoes.

We hope that this list is incomplete. After calling every catalog and large size store in the nation we knew, such a short list is disappointing! Tell your local large size clothing or department store what you need. With all of our voices (and dollars) together, maybe they will listen harder!

Sewing Information
Patterns

Butterick
161 6th Ave.
New York, NY 10013
(800) 221-2670
  Dance and activewear patterns to 46″ hips.

Great Fit Patterns
221 S.E. 197th Ave.
Room G86
Portland, OR 97233
(503)665-3125
  Sportswear patterns, sizes 38–60.

Kwik-Sew
3000 Washington Ave. N.
N. Minneapolis, MN 55422
(800) 328-3953
  Multi-size activewear patterns to 45″ hips. $3 catalogue.

McCall's
230 Park Ave.
New York, NY 10169
(212) 880-2600
  Leotard and activewear patterns to 48″ hips.

Simplicity
200 Madison Ave.
New York, NY 10017
(800) 223-1664
Pattern for warm-ups to 50″ hips.

Stretch & Sew (c/o
Stretch & Sew Fabrics)
Valley River Dr.
Eugene, OR 97401
(503) 686-9263
Materials and books to help you
create activewear:
"Sew You're Not a Size 12" ($4.95);
"Easy Fit"

($5.95); "Get Physical" ($1.00); "Sew
Splashy"
($5.95). Shipping $2 1st item, $.50/additional item.
Knits, cotton, nylon, lycra.

Vogue
161 6th Ave.
New York, NY 10013
(800) 221-2670
Dancewear patterns to 42″ hips.

Leslie Fogel
5 South Molton Street,
London, W1Y 1DHY,
Tel (01) 493 2541.

Fabrics

Fabric Cut-Aways
P.O. Box 292
Glendale, SC 29346
$.50 catalogue. Fabric by the piece, the
pound, or the yard. Velours, sweatshirting, nylon, lycra, and T-shirting.

Fabrics by Mail
Bead Different
1627 S. Tejon
Colorado Springs, CO 80906
(303) 473-2188

Fabrics for dancers and skaters: solids,
prints in cotton, nylon, lycra. Send business-sized SASE for free information.

Stretch & Sew (c/o
Stretch & Sew Fabrics)
Valley River Dr.
Eugene, OR 97401
(503) 686-9263
Cotton- and nylon-Lycra blends, knits, t-
and sweatshirting.

References

Sewing Activewear Video $34.95
Nancy's Notions, Ltd.   3.00 shipping/handling
P.O. Box 683
Beaver Dam, WI 53916 $20.00 to rent tape for two weeks
(414) 885-9175

Brown, Gail, "1-2-3 Aerobicwear!" *It's Me Magazine,* vol. 5, #1,
January–February, 1985, pp. 26–28.

Appendix IV

Becoming an Instructor

If you are considering teaching a class yourself, all of the considerations in Chapter 3 (Hiring an Instructor) apply, only now it will be you making those decisions. Reread that section of the book first, then come back to this point. How do you tell if you're ready to teach a class?

- Assess your knowledge about exercise and fitness. Do you have a good working idea of how your muscles fit together to move?

- Some of us have studied yoga, some have taken too many exercise classes to count, some have academic knowledge about anatomy and exercise physiology, others have studied dance. The decision about when you have enough knowledge to teach is tricky, and even more so in this situation because science knows so little about what pertains specifically to teaching larger, heavier people. Using this book and the others listed in the appendix can be a start. There might be someone who is already an instructor who would be willing to coach and train you.

- Ultimately, it is a personal, ethical decision, and the major criterion for making it is whether you are going to be a benefit or a hazard to your students. If you are a larger person you have the advantage of being able to use your own body for feedback as you teach—to make decisions on pace, selecting exercises, and so on. But be exquisitely sensitive to your students and demand that they tell you how they're feeling. Also demand that they take responsibility for monitoring their exertion level and physical comfort. I have found that people are more able to stop when they need to or challenge themselves when they need to when I frequently remind them of that choice and build it in to what we're doing. For example, I will demonstrate the form of an exercise that requires the minimum of effort and only then say, "For those of you who want more of a challenge, do this." It means that the people who are exerting themselves *more* are the deviant ones rather than the typical situation where the people who can't keep up have to "drop out" and feel like failures.

♦ Take the Red Cross training in CPR (cardiopulmonary resuscitation) in your area and, if you're even more inspired, in first aid.

♦ Join AFAA (The Aerobic and Fitness Association of America) and become certified. AFAA is currently the only organization with a special certification for teaching large people. Once you have a primary certification in aerobics, you are eligible to take the 2-day specialty program. For information, write to: Fitness for the Overweight, AFAA, 15250 Ventura Blvd., Suite 310, Sherman Oaks, CA 91403 or call (800) 445-5950 (outside California), (800) 3-HEALTH (within California).

♦ Go to as many other exercise and dance classes as you can (taking care of yourself as you go!) for "continuing education." You will find both positive new ideas and negative practices that you can critique as your knowledge grows.

♦ *On leadership:* When you first start teaching, you might find it strange to be telling people what to do for an entire hour. It takes some time to get used to hearing yourself talk constantly! But people look to you for the structure of the class, and it's your job to provide it. This means explaining and demonstrating an exercise, then doing it in a rhythmic, easy-to-follow way with your class or getting them started and then making the rounds of the room to offer corrections where necessary. I speak as a dancer when I exhort you to time your exercise's repetitions with the music and save your shifts for shifts in the music! It makes it much easier for your students to give themselves over to the music when you don't conflict with it.

♦ Speaking of *music,* you will need to decide how you are going to produce it. If you can afford live musicians, they are delightful! But most of us will use recorded music, either records or tapes. I have found tapes more useful, requiring fewer interruptions and less extensive stereo equipment. I carry my own little system around with me, a cassette player that hooks up to two portable speakers. Some spaces you will consider may have their own sound systems, but many more places, including churches and schools, become suitable for classes when you can provide the sound equipment they lack. If you make a tape, remember to select appropriate music for each stage of your workout, from warm-up to cool-down and everything in between. It's good to make several tapes so your students don't become tired of hearing the same music over and over.

♦ There are at least two ways to *choreograph a song* for aerobic dance. One is to come up with three or four steps and do each one for a while throughout the song. The second is to "diagram" the song into its component parts and associate a step with each part. Each method has its advantages: Sometimes it's easier for students to learn when you always do the step the same number of times; on the other hand, you're really dancing to the music with the second method.

You could use any of the steps shown in Chapter 5 to compose a sequence using the first method. Try them out with the music. It should feel right; for example, if the musical phrase is only four beats, a sixteen-beat step may not fit. Also, pay attention to the transitions between steps. Is it a smooth change to go from the last movement in one to the first in another? On which foot does each step start? It's easier to learn if it's always on one side, but it gives you a lopsided workout that way.

To use the second method, get a paper and pencil before putting on the music. Label your notes: introduction, verse, bridge, chorus, solo, and so forth. Then count your way through the song. I usually record a tally mark for each set of eight beats. In most songs the song parts have different lengths. For example, the verse may have four sets of eight beats the first time around but only two sets in the third cycle. Or there may be a bridge in between the verse and the chorus in the first cycle but not in the second. In any case, the length of time you do the associated step will vary with the length of the song part.

♦ On the thorny issue of *insurance* and *lawsuits,* different places have different policies. You may have to have your students sign a form stating that they understand you (and/or the studio) do not provide insurance coverage for any accidents and that they understand and assume any risks in participating in the class. If you are responsible in providing a safe place free of hazards, and informing and getting consent from your students, you will be doing what you can to protect yourself. For more detailed information about this constantly shifting issue and the specific laws in your state, you should consult an attorney.

◆   How about *publicity*? If you offer your class through the Y or another established place, they may do your publicity for you or at least foot the bill. Otherwise, you'll need to prepare flyers and maybe a small display ad to run in local publications. Think of a catchy name and choose a good picture or graphic that will grab people. Additionally, there are many sources of *free* publicity:

> ◆ Post your announcement/flyer in churches; large-size clothing shops, hairdressers' and alteration shops, laundromats, and so forth. I have purposely avoided recruiting people at dieting centers since my class is not oriented toward weight loss, but you may have no objections to doing so.
> ◆ Contact physicians and nutritionists, who can be good for referrals.
> ◆ Engage your local media in the excitement of what you're doing. Newspaper reporters and radio and TV talk-show hosts are all looking for a good story, and these classes make good copy.
> ◆ Many newsletters and local papers have "calendar" sections that will run your schedule and information for free.
> ◆ Your local chapter of The National Association to Advance Fat Acceptance (NAAFA) may be willing to publicize your efforts.
> ◆ Put an ad in *Radiance* magazine or *Big Beautiful Woman* that will tell others about your new class. See the appendix for the addresses.

Finally: *Be patient!* It takes a while for news to travel and for a strong core group to form a consistent class. It also takes time for you to evolve your own workout format, your own style. But it is so worth it!

Appendix V

For Instructors: Starting a Class for Large Women

If you are already teaching exercise or aerobics classes and are curious about how to expand your program to include large women, don't miss the suggestions in Appendix IV. More broadly there are two fundamental issues to consider: physical safety and psychological safety.

Physical Safety

The fact that large women are carrying more weight means they are doing more physical work with each movement than their average-size sisters. You need to slow down the pace of your aerobics segment and eliminate any high-impact movements. In We Dance, the aerobic movements are very much like "going out to dance" kind of dancing; the stroll, the Charleston, the pony, and so on. I choreograph one step for each part of the song so that there's a step for the chorus, a different one for the verse, and so forth. When the music changes, we change, so we're dancing to the music. You will probably find that these people can get their heart rate into the aerobic range doing movements that are smoother and slower than what you use in your other classes.

Make sure your floor has lots of give to it. Even if you teach a low-impact class, it's good for people to wear shoes—provided they fit. Many large women have wide feet, and they may find that men's aerobic shoes fit better across the ball of the foot; unfortunately, men's shoes are often loose around the heel. As we go to press, AVIA is coming out with a low-impact women's shoe but only in medium widths. There's no perfect solution yet.

In doing floor work, focus on strengthening the abdominals and the legs. Many students will have a history of back and knee problems, and some will exhibit various degrees of misalignment, such as knock-knees, hyperextended knees, supination, or pronation. The floor work should strengthen the weak muscles and stretch the tight muscles (see Judy Alter's books, *Surviving Exercise* and *Stretch and Strengthen,* for safe exercises). The exercises should be possible to do correctly even with big thighs or a large stomach. Don't ask your students to choose between breathing and doing the exercise right! And remember that your student is lifting body parts that weigh more than yours. She can make the movement smaller and do fewer repetitions and build the same degree of strength.

It's not clear from the scanty research on this subject whether this group of people is at a greater medical risk in doing exercise than average-size students when the class is geared for them. In the best of all possible worlds, your students would have access to inexpensive, compassionate medical care that included safely administered treadmill tests. But most people are probably not going to get much sound information about how their body will react to aerobic exercise. You can ask, for your own information, about the following:

- family history of heart disease
- hypertension
- diabetes
- arthritis
- past or current injuries
- smoking
- dieting history (dramatic weight swings and frequent use of low-calorie diets may leave the heart in a weakened condition)
- birth control pills and other substance use

You might want to consult with a medical specialist or a physical therapist. The problem is that there is conflicting advice about obesity and exercise, with most medical practitioners advising their patients to get more exercise but others cautioning about its hazards. All you can do is make your class as safe as possible, learn CPR, and demand from your students that they become a partner with you in deciding when to push ahead and when to back off. Teach them the difference between muscle fatigue and pain, and make it easy for them to take care of themselves. For example, most instructors tell their students to go at their own pace and hope that each person has the strength of character to deviate from the rest of the class when necessary. It rarely happens. Therefore, I usually lead the class in the easiest form of an exercise, then say, "For those of you who want more of a challenge, do this," so that it's the students who want to work harder who have to make an active choice to deviate. That seems to make it easier for those students who shouldn't be working so hard to honor their own pace.

Psychological Safety

Probably the central issue of psychological safety is whether the class serves to repeat the unpleasant experiences of the past or whether it opens up new possibilities for self-acceptance. Most of these women have been on diets, have been told to lose weight, have been cajoled, prodded, nagged, and harassed to death. They will arrive at the class with an agenda to lose weight, and pronto; and they will expect to be treated the same as they always have—which is to say poorly. And if they are, they will respond by leaving and feeling that they've failed again.

So how do you give them a different experience? In We Dance I never talk about weight loss. The fact is that no one has a method for people to permanently lose large amounts of weight. If someone did, everyone would do it and that would be that. The most you can do is give people an experience of physical activity that is safe and fun so they will come back for more. If movement becomes a permanent part of their lives, they will become healthier from the exercise alone, regardless of whether they lose weight. They will experience doing something for the intrinsic pleasure of it rather than for how they will look from the outside. And they will begin overcoming the terrible social isolation that large people face in this fat-hating culture.

One basic method of providing a psychologically safe place for large women is to restrict the class. We Dance is exclusively for women over two hundred pounds, which is an admittedly arbitrary cutoff point. Most of these women have had the experience of being the largest person wherever they were and of continually feeling huge and distorted. To be around other women their own size is a very healing experience.

It is important that the class be visually private, without on-lookers. Studios that combine the exercise space and the weight room are undesirable unless the people working out with weights are also large women. Most women prefer a sex-segregated class, but if you have the time and space, you could offer one class for women and one coed class to satisfy more people's needs.

If it is possible, you should time the class so that your students can arrive and leave without running into a group of thin women. A buffer zone of half an hour before and after your class is ideal.

After a while the women in the class will get to know one another and form a social network, exchanging information on medical doctors who are caring and competent; where to buy large leotards and tights; good books; other activities for large women; and so on. This is a very exciting development because the class can serve as a catalyst for all kinds of expanded opportunities for its students.

Finally, an instructor who is large herself is a wonderful source of inspiration and psychological safety to the students. The ideal instructor is someone who knows exercise physiology; teaches in a competent, smooth manner; and is capable of communicating her own joy in moving to the class. If she is a large woman who is at peace with her body, she can serve as an inspiration to her students, encouraging them to enjoy the experience of the class as an end in itself rather than as a means to weight loss or as a punishment to endure for being fat. This is important because after the short-term motivation to lose weight wears off for your students, the motivation to experience that kind of physical pleasure and psychological seren-ity is what keeps them coming back.

Finding Your Students

How do you market your class? There are two magazines for large women in which you should consider advertising: *Radiance*

(415) 482-0680 and *Big Beautiful Woman* (available at newsstands). It doesn't cost much to advertise in the Yellow Pages (about $25 a month), and if there are large-size clothing stores in your area, they are the best place to post a flyer or offer coupons. Consider a "community events" listing in your local paper, a notice in a church bulletin, flyers at the grocery, and so forth. After a while word-of-mouth will bring you the most students. This is a group of people who are ready and raring to go, given the opportunity.

It will be the people who are most active and self-accepting already who will have the courage to try out your class. But remember that no matter how good your class is, it will not meet everyone's needs. This group of people has movement preferences that are as varied as those of any other group. Some will find your class too dance-oriented; others, not enough. Some will love your music, others will hate it. And so on. Most of the people who hear about your class will not call you for information; most of the people who call will never show up; and most of the people who come to the class will not become regulars. This is the nature of the situation—your class will be a new idea, and it will take time for people to accept it. If we want our students to make a permanent change rather than yet another failed attempt to get a "quick fix," we have to refrain from the prodding, nagging, cajoling style of teaching and allow them their fits and starts. People call when they are ready; they show up to check it out when they are ready; and they become regulars when they are ready. Paradoxically, the less you evidence an agenda of your own for people to come to class, the more willing they will be to come.

Teaching a class like this demands a certain level of commitment. It takes time for a core group of students to develop; it takes effort to find a larger instructor who is competent and exuberant; it takes a good time slot with buffer zones before and after so that larger students are not comparing themselves to the thin ones; it takes a willingness on the instructor's part to examine how she feels about her own body and what she communicates to these women and to learn from her students about the best way to teach them. If you are willing to make such a commitment, the rewards are significant. You are providing a safe environment for people who often have an adversarial relationship with their bodies to make peace with themselves and have some fun. You are planting the notion that every body deserves the pleasure of physical movement and a sense of competence and grace.

At the risk of sounding too Californian, we urge you to examine your own heart. If your motivation is to reshape all these people into genetically thin folks, you will fail. But if you want to give them an arena where they can explore and play and learn, you have our best wishes. Good luck!

Index

abdominal muscles 76, 173
accessibility
  clothes that fit 21–22
activities
  listings 199–204
aerobic exercise 41, 43
  determining proper duration 93
  for cardiovascular fitness 43
  for strength building 42
Aerobic Fitness Association of America (AFAA) 56
aerobic wear
  see clothing
alignment
  postural 76, 85, 87, 232
Alter, Judy 56, 67 173
Amateur Softball Association 131
American College of Sports Medicine (ACSM) 56
American Indian 23, 140
American lifestyle 18
Ample Opportunity 117
anaerobic exercise 41
anger 170
anorexics 38
athletic clubs 139
athletic scholarships 139
attitude 29–30, 135

back problems 173
balance 11, 154
  of opposing muscle groups 76

barriers 18–24, 168
Bay to Breakers 4, 111
behavior 31, 32
Bennett, William 37, 40
Benoit, Joan 127
Berkman/Syme, 1979 15
bicycling 139
  books recommended 191
bioelectrical impedance 42
biological weight 38
body awareness 47, 145–67
  recommended books 194
body fat percentage 42
body hatred 146
body image 127, 160
Boutilier, Mary 133
breathing 46–7, 154, 156
  and abdominal exercises 78–9
  importance of 47
  while swimming 118
Brody, Jane 39
buddy 33

calipers 42
calisthenics
  and body shape 46–7
  history of 130
cardiac stress test 50
cardiovascular fitness 44
  maintaining 44

chafing 106
change 169
  short- and long-term 26
  permanent vs. short-term 169
check-up, medical 49–50
chest pain 112
child care 20
childhood
  establishing skills 18
  taking physical risks 19
children
  sedentary 18
Cinderella myth 16
City Sports magazine 133
classes
  locating 54–5
  organizing 55–6
clothing 51–4
  bras 52
  catalogues
  criteria for selection 51–4
  exercise 21–2
  layering 106
  listing of outlets 217–225
  mail order 217–225
  suppliers 217–225
coaching 148, 164
comeback 166–8
commitment
  to exercise 20
competition 132–35, 153
concentration 149, 153
concerns 29–30
controlled movement 76
cool-down 58–74, 99–100, 173
  definition 59
  for walking 102–3
cosmetics industries 21
cost
  of regular exercise 19–20
couch-potato syndrome 18
Court, Margaret 131
Cousins, Norman 17
CPR 56
cultural expectations 177–8
cycling 140

dancewear, see clothing
De Beauvior, Simone 134
depression 7, 15

deviation from others 47
dieting 9, 12
  cycles 12
  history of 193
  and setpoint 39
  side effects of 41
  vs. exercise as weight loss treatment 41
  yo-yo cycle 9
discomfort 176
doctors 49–50
  and fat-phobic attitudes 49

eating disorders
  recommended books 194–5
effort vs. visualization 154–5
elite training 142
embarrassment 169
encouragement 19
  importance of 18
energy
  conserving during dieting 38
exercise
  aerobic 41
  anaerobic 41
  concerns for large bodies 45–6
  as a duty 11
  and family member reaction 174–5
  as healing 28
  for large bodies 36
  starting positions for 61
  vs. dieting 41
  and weight 36–57
  and weight change 42
exercises
  calves 69–71
  cool-down 61–74
  hamstrings 69–71
  heels 69–71
  hips 68
  neck 62–64
  shoulder 64–6
  strengthening 77–93
  torso 66–8
  transition steps 73–4
  warm-up 61–74
exercise classes
  listings 199–204

fat and fit 24
Fat Chance 2

fat fitness books 189–90
Fat Underground 16
fear 29
    realistic and unrealistic 174
feelings 28
femininity
    and athletics 128, 132
first aid 48, 174
fitness for large women, books 190
fluids 98
    maintaining during exertion 48
    and swimming 122
    and walking 105
football 165
Friends Are Good Medicine campaign
    15

Gallwey, Tim 150
Garrick, Dr. James 48
goals 30–35
    reachable 30
Greendorder, Susan 18
guilt 174–5
Gurin, Joel 37

harassment 140
health 6, 21
    source of beauty 21
health care practitioners
    criteria for selection 49–50
heart rate
    and fitness level 100
heat exhaustion 106
heredity
    and setpoint 39
hiking 113–14, 123–25
    supplies 114
humiliation 169–71
hunger to move 26, 29

impact 112
    injuries 46
    transforming high to low 46
injury 103
    and body weight 174
    fear of 172–74
Inner Game 146, 150
instructor
    auditioning 55–6

becoming an 227
body size of 55, 179
and leadership 228
movement styles of an 55
teaching large people 231–35
insurance liability 229
internal awareness
    and walking 156–61
International Dance-Exercise Association (IDEA)
    56
isolation 14, 16
isolation exercises
    purpose of 76

joints 173
    hyperextending 100
    overbending 100

karate 138
King, Billie Jean 131
knees
    and exercise modifications 89
Kriegel, Bob 153
Kuntzleman, Charles 106

lactic acid 48, 76
large
    defining 116–17
Leonard, George 127
lifestyle
    American 18
    sedentary 18
ligaments 100
low-impact activities 46, 99

magazines and newsletters 196
martial arts 138
medical advice 49
mental imaging 163
metabolism 38
miracle cure 21
model mugging 110–11
motivation 168–88
motivational testimonies 182–86
muscle fatigue 233
muscle fiber 135
muscles
    and daily routine 76

music 56
myth
    of exercise as a cure-all 181

National Association to Advance Fat Acceptance
    (NAAFA) 14, 50
Nautilus 138
normal eating 40
North American Network of Women Runners
    109
Nyad, Diana 144

Oakland Raters 101
Olympic games 128
organizations 205–6
overexertion 46
    signs of 112
overfeeding 38

pain
    distinguishing types of 112–13
    emotional 176
    evaluating dangers of 47–8
PE teachers 134
people-pleasing 31
perfect body 134
physical activity
    of daily life 26
    degrees of 31–2
physical examination 172
physical safety 45, 109, 231
physical therapy 176
plateauing 39
pre-exercise medical evaluation 50
preferences for activities 26–7
prejudice 14
preparation 170
pronation 54
psychological safety 233
publicity 230
pulse 92, 99
    locating 43
    resting 43
    recovery 43

Radiance magazine 13
Radiance Retreat 13, 17, 176
range of motion 77
rebellion 25
recess 13, 17, 187–88

recovery pulse 43
relaxation exercise 26–7
repetitions 76
research
    recommended books 197
resistance 77
respect 23
resting pulse 43
Riggs, Bobby 131
right to exercise 1, 178, 188
risks 19
running 111–12
    books recommended 191
    transition from walking 112

San Giovanni, Lucinda 133
Satter, Ellyn 16
sedentary 18
segregation 55, 116
self acceptance 148
self awareness 153, 167
self contempt 25–6
self criticism 136, 147, 167
self defense 110–11
self discovery vs. self improvement 186
self improvement 178, 188
self respect 23
setpoint
    determining 40
    and dieting 39
    and environmental factors 39
    and exercise 41
    setting 39, 41
setpoint theory 37–9
shame 169
shoes 52–54, 112
    criteria for selection 52
    designed for specific activities 53
    importance of 52
    for running 52–4
    for walking 52–4
social prejudice 16
social support 15
sociology of body size
    recommended books 193
softball 165
sports 126–44
    aerobics vs. non-aerobics 137, 143–4
    and militarism 130
    selection and body weight 136

and weight loss agenda 133
and winning 132
sports psychology 124, 145–67
books recommended 192
spot reduction 75
starting position
for warm-ups or stretching 61
starvation 37–8
mode 39
response 41
stiffness 176
stretch and strengthen
principle of 190–91
strength building
using water resistance 119–20
stretch reflex 60
stretches 58–74
stretching
after exertion 59
ballistic 60
importance of 59, 173
purpose of 59–60, 100
for walking 103
success
barometers of 187
supinaiton 54
surfaces 104
sweating 106
swimming 114–123
and body fat 119
and breathing 118
equipment 121
lap 117, 120
open water 122
organized 115
synchronized 117, 122
swimming instruction 120
swimming pools 115
swimsuits 120–21

talk test 44, 107, 112
target heart rate 42–3, 44, 93, 107, 112,
122
subjectively determined 44
teaching 231
team sports 141
tendons 173
time 19–20
required to exercise regularly 19–20
Title IX federal legislation 131

training routine 143
treadmill tests 50
Twin, Stephanie 129
"Type A" personality 137

UCSF Study (1986) 12
Ullyot, Joan 111
underwater (hydrostatic) weighing 42
unitard, definition 50
unsolicited advice 7

video
listings 206–15
ratings 206–15
visualization 161–53
of sports techniques 162–63
volleyball
in swimming pool 123

walking 101–14, 191
accessibility of 102
arm swing 108
companionship 108
and internal awareness 156–61
and postural alignment 107
routes to take 109
safety 109
in shopping malls 102, 106
in swimming pool 120
tips 104
transition to running 112
Walking magazine 102
warm-up 58–74
definition 59
importance of 173
purpose 58
for walking 102–3
water 106
water ballet 117
We Dance 14, 33, 49, 75
exercises 75–93
We Dance Steps 94–100
box step 97
charleston 94
rocking step 99
the stroll 96
weather conditions 106
weight charts 23, 38
weight lifting 137–38

weight loss 10
weight loss industry 21
weight loss surgery 9
Weight Watchers 17
willpower 25–6, 39
women in sports
    history of 127–35

women's sports
    recommended books 192
Women's Sports Foundations 131
Women's Sports magazine 131
Wooley, Susan 8

yo-yo cycle 9, 40

Printed in the United States
41612LVS00005B/48